Disorders of Cardiac Rate, Rhytl.... and Conduction

Hamish Watson

MD, FRCP, FACC

Postgraduate Dean and Director of Postgraduate Medical Education
Chairman, Section of Cardiology, Department of Medicine
University of Dundee, Scotland

Consultant Cardiologist, Tayside Area, Scotland

BEACONSFIELD PUBLISHERS LTD
Beaconsfield, Bucks, England

This book is dedicated to Rae Gilchrist,
teacher, colleague and friend

First published in 1984

British Library Cataloguing in Publication Data
Watson, Hamish
    Disorders of cardiac rate, rhythm and conduction.
    1. Cardiovascular system—Diseases
    I. Title
    616.1   RC667

ISBN 0-906584-10-8

Phototypeset by Prima Graphics, Camberley, Surrey
in 11 on 12 and 10 on 11 point Times.
Printed in Great Britain at the University Press, Oxford.

Preface

Recent developments in monitoring the electrocardiogram have demonstrated that disorders of rate, rhythm and conduction are so common that many of them can now almost be regarded as a normal occurrence. They are no longer the preserve of cardiologists and physicians with an interest in heart disease and, although some of the more serious disorders still require specialist attention, many of those that are relatively benign can easily be diagnosed and treated by the general practitioner without recourse to outside assistance.

This book is written as a practical guide for the non-specialist. It begins with the necessary background information on electrophysiology and the way in which normal and abnormal conditions are displayed on the ECG. It then discusses the symptoms associated with disorders of rate, rhythm and conduction, and patients who have no symptoms. This is followed by a major section on recognition and treatment, dealing in turn with variations of normal sinus rhythm, disorders of rate and rhythm, and disorders of conduction. The next section contains a selection of drugs and physical methods, with detailed information on their use and possible side effects. The final section comprises three groups of six fictitious management problems, written respectively for general practitioners, hospital doctors and nurses. The patient's problem is presented and the reader is asked to make decisions about diagnosis, further investigation and management.

At each stage of the problem, reference is made to the relevant part of the explanatory text, and the author also states what in his view is the most appropriate decision. The reader can either work through the main part of the text to acquire an overview of the subject, or else start with the problems and refer to the text as necessary. Afterwards, the book will be of value in the practical management of clinical cases.

The drugs selected are all of proved value. None have been included that are considered to be still under clinical trial. The suggested doses are offered only as guidelines, subject in every case to the user's clinical judgement and the manufacturer's current recommendations. To avoid confusion, the pharmacopoeial or non-proprietary as well as proprietary names have been given in the section on Treatment.

Throughout the problem-solving exercises, doctors are referred to as 'he' and nurses as 'she'. This convention is used for simplicity and is in no way meant to disparage the contributions of my female medical and male nursing colleagues.

The project was originally conceived with Professor R. M. Harden and Mr W. R. Dunn as a distance-learning course for general practitioners. It soon became clear that it fulfilled a need; and not only for those engaged in primary care. The present book has developed out of our experience with the earlier version. The contributions and support of Professor Harden and Mr Dunn are gratefully acknowledged, as are those of Dr G. P. McNeill, Dr M. D. Clee, Dr J. C. Murdoch, Dr Norma Smith, Mrs Cynthia Stone, Mrs Suzette Sowden, Miss Maureen Sneddon and Mrs Elsie Jeffrey. The text has been extensively revised and rearranged in preparation for its publication in book form, and I am indebted to Miss Audrey Gibson, Mrs Joyce Strachan and Miss Gail Stout for helping me to do this. Also, to Mr John Churchill of Beaconsfield Publishers Ltd, who has given such enthusiastic support during its metamorphosis.

H. W.

Contents

1
BACKGROUND INFORMATION

As the management of patients with disorders of rate, rhythm and conduction varies from reassurance, through simple or complex drug therapy, to DC cardioversion, intracardiac pacing or even, in rare instances, cardiac surgery, a basic knowledge of a few electrophysiological and pharmacological principles is essential for anyone who is considering the most appropriate measures to adopt.

Electrophysiology

POLARISATION AND DEPOLARISATION

Rhythmic electrical activity is a characteristic of all myocardial cells. Most of them are electrically stable at rest when the intracellular potassium is high and the intracellular sodium is low. The cell membrane is negative on the inside and positive on the outside. The difference between these two electrical charges is known as the **transmembrane potential**.

In the resting state, the cell is said to be **polarised**. When the cell membrane is stimulated, sodium ions rush in and potassium ions flow out, with the result that the inside of the cell becomes relatively positive. The cell is then said to be **depolarised**.

THE THRESHOLD POTENTIAL

The electrical stability of each myocardial cell depends upon its **threshold potential (TP)**. This is the level at which, in response to a stimulus, depolarisation becomes self-perpetuating.

REPOLARISATION

Recovery begins almost immediately after depolarisation. Sodium is pumped out and potassium flows back in again. At the end of this recovery phase, the cell is said to be **repolarised**. The cell has returned to its **resting potential (RP)** and remains electrically stable until another stimulus comes along that is powerful enough to overcome its threshold potential.

THE CARDIAC ACTION POTENTIAL

These phases of electrical activity, starting with a polarised cell that becomes depolarised and then repolarised, are collectively referred to as the **cardiac action potential** (Figure 1).

Throughout most of the action potential, the cell cannot be re-excited by another stimulus and is said to be **refractory**. Towards the end of the repolarisation process it is only relatively refractory, but normally, excitability does not return until the membrane potential returns to its intrinsic resting value.

2

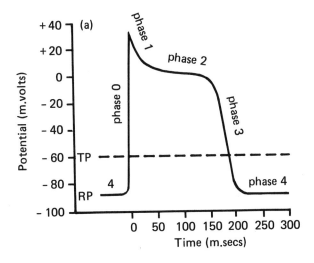

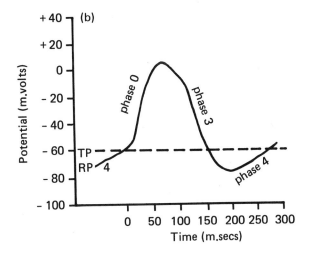

Figure 1. Myocardial cells that do not normally have a pacemaker function are stable at rest and remain so until stimulated. They have a steady resting potential (RP) of about 92mVolts (Figure 1a, phase 4).

When a stimulus lowers the transmembrane potential to its threshold potential (TP), which is usually about 65mVolts, the cell becomes almost instantaneously depolarised (phase 0).

Repolarisation then occurs in three phases:

- an initial rapid phase that corrects the overshoot and returns the transmembrane potential towards zero (phase 1)
- a slow plateau-like phase (phase 2)
- a second and longer rapid phase (phase 3) that restores the cell to its resting potential (phase 4), which it maintains until another stimulus comes along.

Pacemaker cells (Figure 1b) are unstable at rest. They undergo continual spontaneous depolarisation during phase 4. When their threshold potential is reached they become depolarised and this provides the stimulus to the stable myocardial cells. Depolarisation (phase 0) is slower in pacemaker cells than in stable myocardial cells and consequently there is less overshoot. Phases 1 and 2 are less obvious, but phase 3 is well developed.

3

PACEMAKER CELLS

Some cells are unstable at rest. After repolarisation, instead of waiting for the next stimulus to come along, they become **spontaneously depolarised**. This happens because sodium constantly leaks into the cells and raises their transmembrane potential above the threshold level.

These are the **pacemaker cells** of the heart. Their constantly recurring spontaneous depolarisation provides the regular stimuli that excite the stable myocardial cells from their resting state (Figure 2).

The rate of impulse formation and the influence of physiological, pathological and pharmacological factors upon it, is determined by a complex interaction between the speed of spontaneous depolarisation, the level at which the threshold potential is set, the height of maximum depolarisation and the total duration of depolarisation.

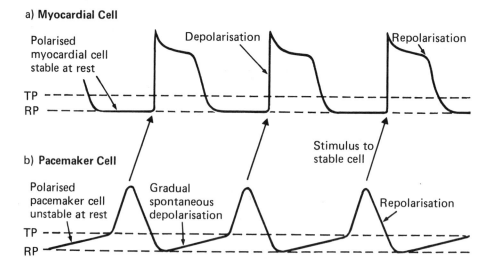

Figure 2. Cardiac action potentials of stable myocardial cells (a) and unstable pacemaker cells (b). Gradual spontaneous depolarisation of the pacemaker cells provides constantly recurring stimuli (diagonal arrows) to the myocardial cells that are stable at rest.

Physiological Pacemakers

In health, pacemaker cells are present in:
- the sinus (SA) node
- the atrioventricular junctional tissues (the AV node and His bundle)
- the right and left bundle branches
- the Purkinje system in the ventricles

4

Each of these has a different **spontaneous depolarisation time**. The shortest time is in the SA node, followed by the AV node, then the bundle of His and finally the Purkinje system.

As a result, each has a different normal **inherent rate of impulse formation:**
- the sinus rate is between 60 and 100 per minute
- the junctional rate is between 40 and 60 per minute
- the Purkinje rate is between 10 and 40 per minute

Physiological and pathological circumstances may cause wide variation from these normal ranges, but their decreasing order of automaticity usually ensures that a lower centre does not normally take over from a higher one.

Sinus Rhythm

The heart is normally dominated by the sinus node. It overrides the activity of all other pacemakers; hence the term **normal sinus rhythm.**

If the sinus node is out of action or less excitable than normal, the next in order takes over the function of pacemaker. This is often referred to as an **escape rhythm**, because the heart has *escaped* from the control of the sinus node.

At normal heart rates the patient is usually unaware of the change as one pacemaker takes over from another. At faster rates, if a potential pacemaker in the atrial, junctional or ventricular tissues fires more rapidly than the prevailing sinus rate, it will initiate a tachycardia and may cause symptoms.

Pathological Pacemakers

In addition to these natural pacemakers, any myocardial cell may lose its electrical stability at rest, take upon itself the role of an **ectopic pacemaker**, and initiate an ectopic rhythm. Such rhythms are common in the presence of clinically recognisable heart disease, but may also occur in the absence of demonstrable cardiac pathology.

AUTOMATICITY, CONDUCTIVITY AND EXCITABILITY

Automaticity is the capacity of a cell to originate an impulse. **Conductivity** is the ability of a cell to propagate an impulse. **Excitability** is the property that permits a cell to respond to an impulse. Automaticity, conductivity and excitability may be influenced by many physiological, pathological and pharmacological factors.

Physiological factors include:
- sympathetic and parasympathetic activity
- circulating catecholamines
- electrolyte and acid/base balance
- temperature and stretch

Pathological factors include:
- ischaemia, inflammation, infiltrative and collagen diseases
- abnormalities of development
- surgical treatment

Pharmacological factors include the effects of a wide range of drugs on:
- the myocardium
- the cardiac action potential

Any of these factors may be of major importance in the aetiology and treatment of the disorders of rate, rhythm and conduction encountered in daily practice. Although automaticity, conductivity and excitability are often similarly affected, this is not necessarily so. One may be affected more than the others or they may be affected differently. For example, toxic doses of digitalis may enhance automaticity, but depress conductivity and excitability.

THE CONDUCTION SYSTEM

The conduction system (Figure 3) is developed at a very early stage in the growth of the embryonic heart from specially differentiated muscle fibres. Its function is to initiate and conduct impulses that maintain and co-ordinate atrial and ventricular contractions to ensure an adequate output.

It consists of:
- the sinus (SA or sino atrial) node
- the atrioventricular (AV) node
- the atrioventricular bundle (of His)
- the left and right bundle branches
- a network of Purkinje fibres in the ventricular walls

The sinus node lies in the upper part of the lateral wall of the right atrium where the root of the right atrial appendage joins the front of the superior vena cava. It has a generous blood supply derived from either the right coronary artery (55%) or the circumflex branch of the left coronary artery (45%).

The AV node lies in the lowest part of the right atrium, just above the opening of the coronary sinus and behind the attachment of the septal cusp of the tricuspid valve. It is usually supplied by a branch from the right coronary artery (90%) or less often from the circumflex branch of the left coronary artery (10%).

Internodal Pathways

Impulses from the SA node spread through the myocardial fibres of the atrial walls to reach the AV node. Special pathways called the anterior, middle and posterior internodal tracts also connect the two nodes, but their exact functions have yet to be determined.

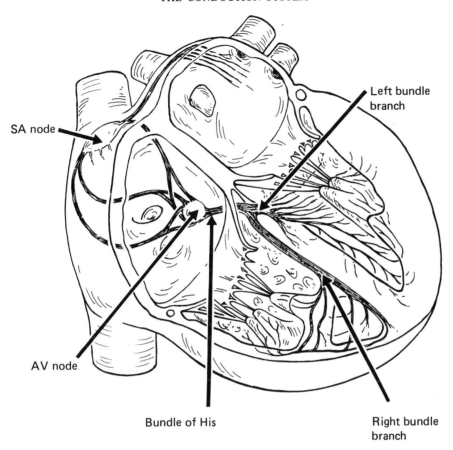

SA node

Left bundle
branch

AV node

Bundle of His

Right bundle
branch

Figure 3. The conduction system.

Junctional Tissues

The AV bundle, which is 2–3cm in length, arises from the lower end of the AV node, the one gradually merging into the other. It bridges the fibrous tissue that separates the atria and the ventricles, and is normally the only connection between the atrial and ventricular myocardium. It traverses the lower margin of the membraneous part of the ventricular septum and divides into left and right branches.

The left bundle branch passes down the left side of the ventricular septum as a thin sheet of fibres and soon splits into two main divisions called the anterior and posterior fascicles. These fan out in the subendocardium to supply the anterosuperior and posterio-inferior parts of the left ventricular myocardium.

The right bundle branch continues down on the right side of the septum and spreads out in the subendocardium to supply all parts of the right ventricle.

Most of the main branches of the AV bundle are supplied by septal branches of the anterior descending branch of the left coronary artery.

7

SPREAD OF THE IMPULSE IN NORMAL CONDUCTION

Impulses arise in the sinus node and spread rapidly through the atrial tissues to produce the **P waves** on the ECG. After activating the atria, they arrive at the AV node, where the rate of conduction is considerably slowed.

This slowing, plus an inherent degree of block that will not accept impulses in too rapid succession, allows adequate time for the ventricles to fill. It produces the **PR interval** on the ECG.

Conduction speeds up again as the impulse passes through the AV bundle, the right and left bundle branches and the ventricular Purkinje fibres. This activates the ventricles and produces the **QRS complexes** on the ECG.

The passage of an impulse may be blocked in the sinus node, the AV node, the AV bundle or the bundle branches.

CAUSES OF ABNORMALITIES OF RATE AND RHYTHM

Three mechanisms are responsible for most abnormalities of rate and rhythm:

1. If the normal pacemaker is more suppressed than a normally subordinate potential pacemaker, or, if a normally subordinate potential pacemaker develops enhanced automaticity, the subordinate pacemaker may take over the pacemaking function and initiate an **escape rhythm**.

2. If a focus that does not normally function as a pacemaker develops a rate of automaticity that is greater than that of the normal pacemaker or any of the potential pacemakers, it may take over the pacemaking function and initiate an **accelerated rhythm**.

3. If unequal refractory periods cause different rates of conduction or unidirectional block to develop in adjacent areas, slow conduction through partially refractory tissue may re-enter and re-activate tissue that has already recovered from faster conduction and initiate an **ectopic rhythm** (Figures 4 and 5). Critical timing is necessary for a stimulus to initiate such circus movement, because, if it arrives too soon, it is blocked and if it arrives too late, it is conducted normally.

The most common **sites of re-entry** are the AV node, the Purkinje/myocardial junctions and areas of ischaemic myocardium.

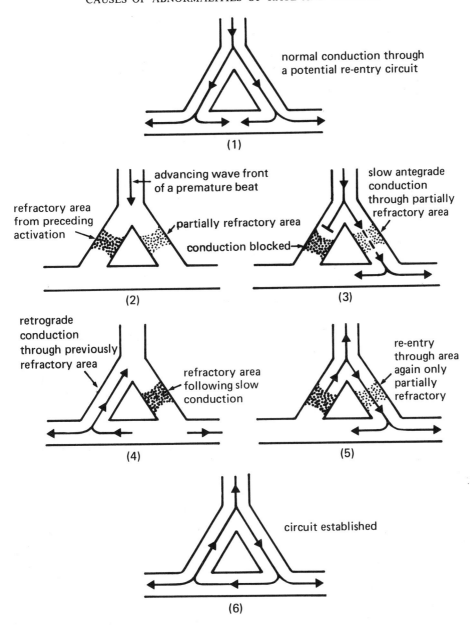

Figure 4. A circuit of re-entry.

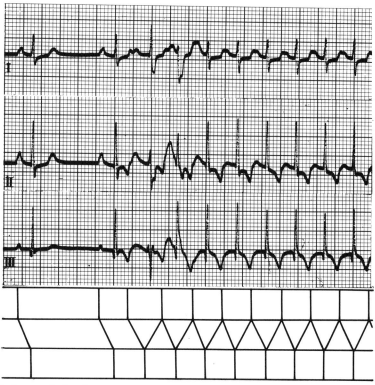

Figure 5. A record showing the onset of re-entrant supraventricular tachycardia. An early ectopic P wave is seen on the upstroke of the T wave of the second normal beat. Coming so soon after the previous cycle, it finds the junctional tissues partially refractory and takes longer to pass through them. The resulting QRS complex is broadened because of aberrant conduction. Having activated the ventricles, the impulse passes back up to reactivate the atria and the circuit becomes complete.

TABLE 1. Heart Rate calculated from the RR Interval (measured in multiples of 0.04 secs (1 small square))

5 = 300 per minute	17 = 88 per minute	34 = 44 per minute
5.5 = 273 per minute	18 = 83 per minute	35 = 43 per minute
6 = 250 per minute	19 = 79 per minute	36 = 42 per minute
6.5 = 231 per minute	20 = 75 per minute	37 = 40 per minute
7 = 214 per minute	21 = 71 per minute	38 = 39 per minute
7.5 = 200 per minute	22 = 68 per minute	40 = 38 per minute
8 = 188 per minute	23 = 65 per minute	42 = 36 per minute
8.5 = 176 per minute	24 = 63 per minute	44 = 34 per minute
9 = 167 per minute	25 = 60 per minute	46 = 33 per minute
9.5 = 158 per minute	26 = 58 per minute	48 = 31 per minute
10 = 150 per minute	27 = 56 per minute	50 = 30 per minute
11 = 136 per minute	28 = 54 per minute	52 = 29 per minute
12 = 125 per minute	29 = 52 per minute	54 = 28 per minute
13 = 115 per minute	30 = 50 per minute	56 = 27 per minute
14 = 107 per minute	31 = 48 per minute	58 = 26 per minute
15 = 100 per minute	32 = 47 per minute	60 = 25 per minute
16 = 93 per minute	33 = 45 per minute	

Interpretation of Electrocardiograms

Electrocardiograms consist of a series of deflections known as P, QRS and T waves that arise from a straight base line known as the iso-electric line. They are usually recorded at 25mm per second on a special paper ruled in 1mm and 5mm squares (Figure 6).

The length of each small square, when expressed as a time interval, is 0.04 seconds or 40 milliseconds. The length of each large square, when expressed as a time interval, is 0.20 seconds or 200 milliseconds.

Nowadays, most ECGs are recorded using machines with a hot stylus that burns a tracing onto a specially treated paper. The quality of the record depends, amongst other things, upon the temperature of the stylus and the magnitude (and consequently the speed) of its deflections from the iso-electric line. If the stylus is not hot enough, large deflections are faintly inscribed and, although adequate for diagnosis, are difficult to reproduce.

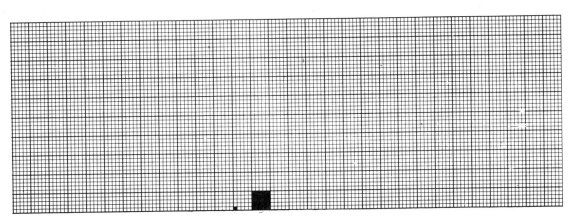

Figure 6.

P waves

P waves are the result of atrial depolarisation and signal atrial contraction. Normally, the right and left atrial P waves are superimposed upon each other so that only one P wave is visible. If left atrial activation is delayed, both may be visible and the deflection becomes M-shaped.

The P waves are usually upright in the standard leads (I, II and III) and should not exceed 0.1 seconds in duration or 3mm in height. Inverted P waves, in leads where they are usually upright, indicate abnormal depolarisation and suggest that the impulse has not arisen in the sinus node.

QRS complexes

The QRS complexes are the result of ventricular depolarisation and signal ventricular contraction. They should not exceed 0.1 second in duration. Their morphology depends upon which ECG lead is being recorded and upon the condition of the conducting tissues and the ventricular myocardium. Broad complexes indicate abnormal depolarisation and suggest defective conduction.

T waves

The T waves are the result of ventricular repolarisation. They follow the QRS complexes and normally point in the same direction because repolarisation of the ventricles takes place in the opposite direction to depolarisation, i.e. from outside inwards, instead of from inside outwards. Their morphology depends largely upon the condition of the myocardium, but is not of much significance when interpreting abnormalities of rate, rhythm and conduction.

ECGs should be studied systematically and the same method should be applied to every record.

RATE

In health, the atrial and ventricular rates are equal and, for practical purposes, the heart rate is the ventricular rate. In abnormalities of rate, rhythm and conduction, the two are not necessarily equal and they must be counted separately.

There are several ways of determining the atrial and ventricular rates. If the rhythm is regular, the most accurate way is to count the small squares between complexes and divide the number into 1500 (the number of small squares in one minute). For convenience, the result can be obtained easily and quickly from a table such as the one shown opposite. If the rhythm is irregular, count the number of complexes recorded on a 15cm strip (30 large squares:6 seconds) and multiply by 10; this will give an approximate rate per minute.

An easier way, if accuracy is not essential, is to use one of the many plastic rulers supplied for the purpose.

RHYTHM AND CONDUCTION

Rhythm and conduction are determined by careful scrutiny of the P, QRS and T waves:
- inspect the 12 lead ECG
- choose a lead where all the deflections are clearly visible (often lead II)
- record a long strip of this lead for analysis

First identify the P waves (arrows) and study their morphology (Figure 7)

Sometimes there are no P waves (Figure 8). Sometimes large fibrillary waves are mistaken for P waves (Figure 9). Sometimes P waves are obscured by the QRST complexes (Figure 10). Sometimes the P waves do not look like ordinary P waves (Figure 11).

12

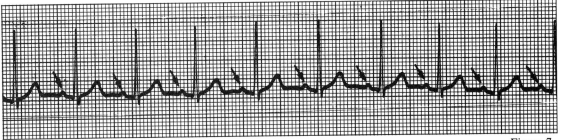

Figure 7.

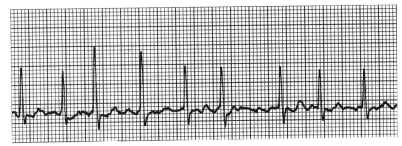

Figure 8. No P waves.

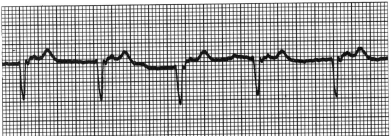

Figure 9. Large fibrillary waves.

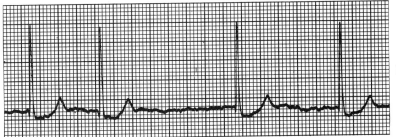

Figure 10. P waves in ST segments.

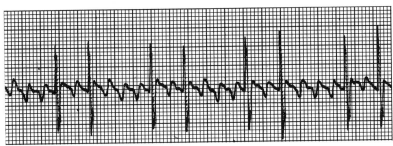

Figure 11. Unusual P waves.

If there are no obvious P waves, pay particular attention to the following, which may give a clue to their whereabouts:
- pauses between QRS complexes (Figure 12)
- notches or irregularities on the QRS and T waves (Figure 13)

Next identify the QRS complexes (arrows) and study their morphology (Fig. 14)

Any supraventricular impulse that is conducted normally through the AV junctional tissues produces a normal QRS complex. Impulses arising in the junctional tissues that are conducted normally to the ventricles also produce 'supraventricular' type QRS complexes, though they may vary slightly from the normal QRS complexes (Figure 15).

Impulses arising in the ventricles (or very low down in the junctional tissues) produce completely different QRS complexes. These are characteristically broad and bizarre, with T waves pointing in the opposite direction to their main deflection. These 'ventricular' type QRS complexes are easily identified (Figure 16), but may sometimes be confused with those showing aberration, which occurs when a supraventricular impulse encounters bundle branch block (Figure 17).

Finally, identify the T waves (arrows) and study their morphology (Figure 18)

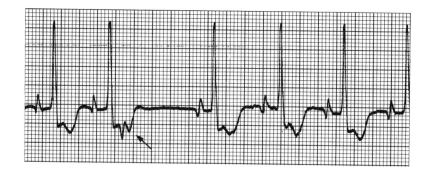

Figure 12. Pauses between QRS complexes.

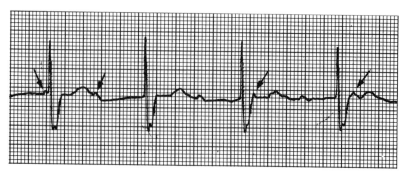

Figure 13. Irregularities on the QRS and T waves.

14

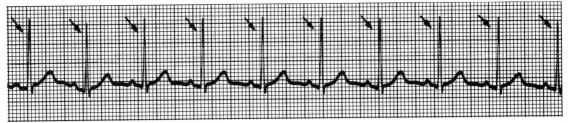

Figure 14.

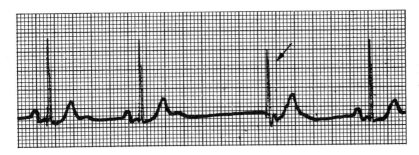

Figure 15.
Junctional escape beat.

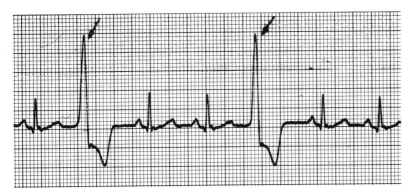

Figure 16.
Ventricular ectopic beats.

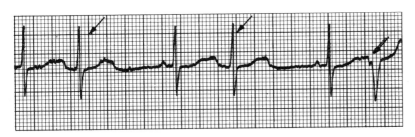

Figure 17. Supraventricular
ectopic beats, the third of
which shows aberrant
conduction.

Figure 18.

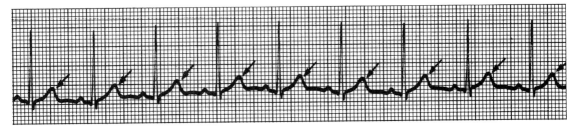

Although the T waves are of relatively little importance in this aspect of electrocardiography, valuable clues about rhythm and conduction can often be detected by careful analysis of the ST-T wave segments (Figures 19 and 20).

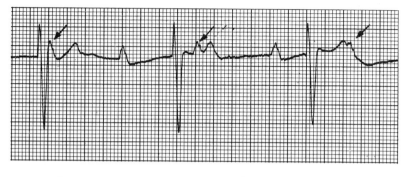

Figure 19. P waves in ST-T wave segments.

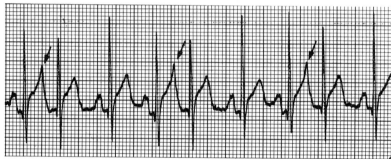

Figure 20. Premature Ps on preceding Ts.

Having identified the various components of the ECG, work out their relationships to one another and to each other.

1. Determine whether or not there is:
(a) a P wave for every QRS complex (Figures 21 and 22).
(b) a QRS complex for every P wave (Figure 23).

2. Measure the PP intervals (the distance between consecutive P waves, Fig. 24) to determine whether or not they are constantly related to one another (Figures 25 and 26).

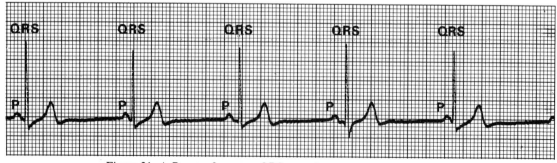

Figure 21. A P wave for every QRS complex.

16

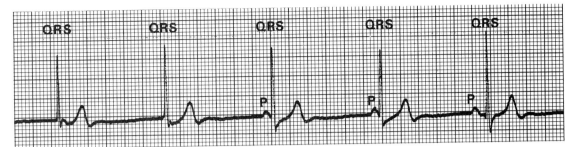

Figure 22. A P wave for only some of the QRS complexes.

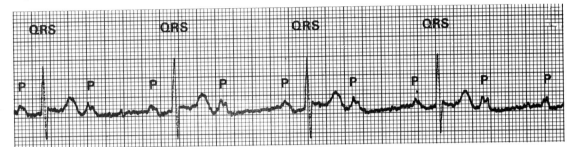

Figure 23. Two P waves for every QRS complex.

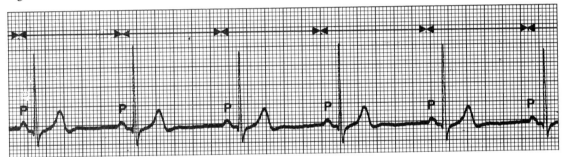

Figure 24. Measure the PP intervals.

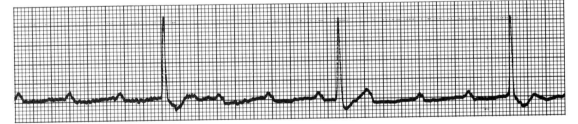

Figure 25. Constantly related Ps.

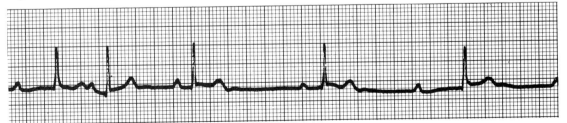

Figure 26. Unrelated Ps.

3. Count the atrial rate.

4. Measure the RR intervals (the distance between consecutive QRS complexes, Figure 27) to determine whether or not they are constantly related to one another (Figures 28 and 29).

5. Count the ventricular rate.

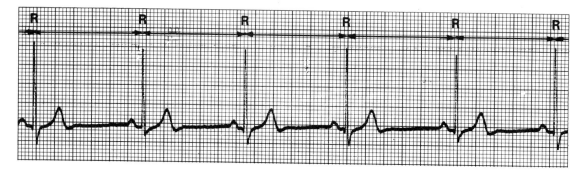

Figure 27. Measure the RR intervals.

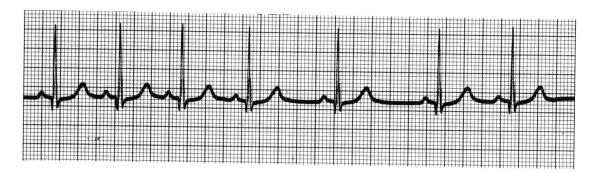

Figure 28. Phasic variation of Rs.

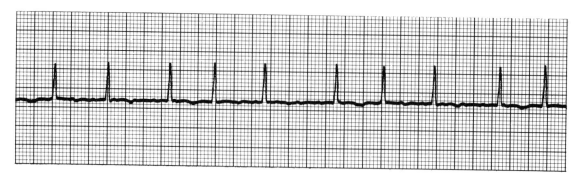

Figure 29. Unrelated Rs.

6. Measure the PR intervals (the distance from the beginning of the P wave to the beginning of the QRS complex, Figure 30) to determine whether or not the P waves and the QRS complexes are constantly related to each other (Figures 31 and 32). This indicates the time taken for the stimulus to activate the atria and pass through the AV junctional tissues to the ventricles. It varies a little with age and heart rate, but in adults it should be between 0.1 and 0.2 seconds.

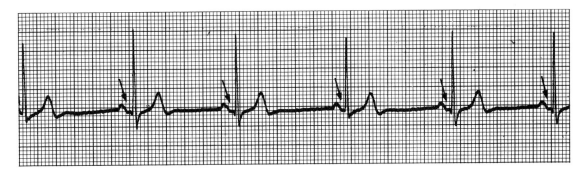

Figure 30. Measure the PR intervals.

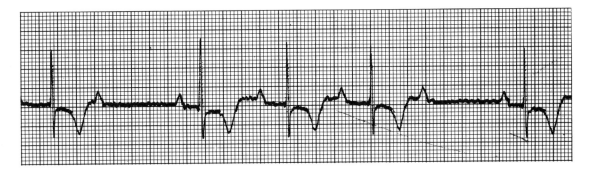

Figure 31. Progressive lengthening of the PR Interval.

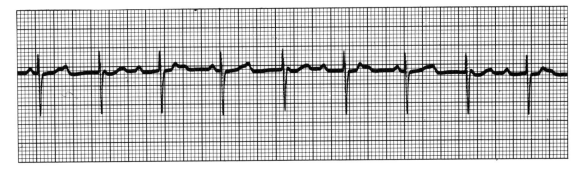

Figure 32. Ps bearing no relationship to the Rs.

Continuous Tape-Recording of ECGs

Tape-recorded ECGs can be of great value in the diagnosis and treatment of disorders of rate, rhythm and conduction; especially those that are paroxysmal, where the chance of catching them on a routine ECG is remote.

If the history is characteristic, as it is in many cases of tachycardia, this is no great problem, but with transient giddy turns or drop attacks, it is essential to know what is happening before, during and after the event. A 24-hour tape will often reveal the cause of the symptoms or indicate that they are not cardiac in origin (Figures 33 and 34).

Carrying a small tape-recorder about presents no difficulty, even to the elderly and infirm, but fitting the electrodes to ensure good quality records requires an experienced technician; as does their analysis, which is both costly and time-consuming. To conserve resources, patients who are thought to require long-term monitoring should be referred to a specialist clinic.

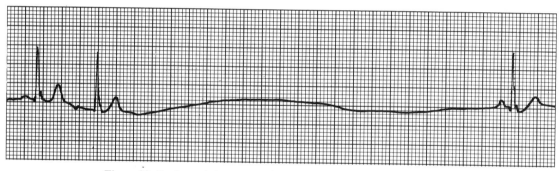

Figure 33. Prolonged sinus arrest in a patient who complained of feeling faint, but in whom no abnormality could be detected.

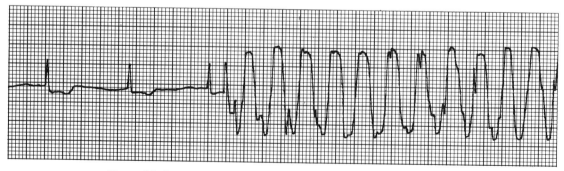

Figure 34. Rapid ventricular tachycardia in a patient who was having blackouts for no apparent reason.

Pacing

Nowadays, many patients have their hearts paced electrically rather than by one of their own pacemakers, and it is necessary to be able to recognise this on the ECG. Also, to be familiar with a few of the more common electrocardiographic signs of pacemaker failure.

The impulse from the battery in the pacemaker is delivered to the heart through an electrode catheter. Being of very short duration (0.5m sec) and of limited strength (5V), it produces a short, sharp, spikey deflection on the ECG known as the **pacing artefact**.

Most pacing catheters make contact with the heart in the apex of the right ventricle, so the impulse does not have to travel through the conducting tissues of the heart. The pacing artefact (arrow) is followed almost immediately by a right ventricular ectopic beat with a broad, bizarre QRS complex (Figure 35).

If, for some reason, the heart fails to respond to the stimulus delivered by the pacemaker, the term 'non-capture' is used. This is recognised on the ECG by pacing artefacts (arrows) that are not followed by QRS complexes (Figure 36).

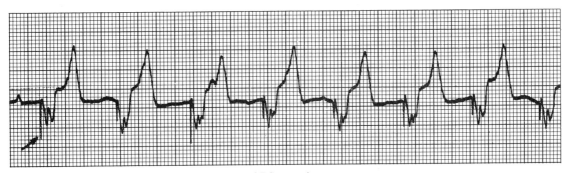

Figure 35. Pacing artefacts (arrow) followed by QRS complexes.

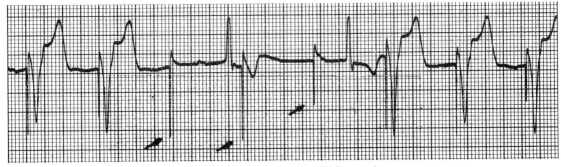

Figure 36. Pacing artefacts (arrows) that are not followed by QRS complexes.

Most pacemakers are of the 'on demand' type. This means that they only function if necessary. They are usually set to discharge around 70 times a minute and do so if the natural heart rate falls below this level (Figure 37).

If the battery in the pacemaker is running down, its discharge rate will fall below that at which it was programmed before insertion. The heart is then driven at the pacemaker's slower rate or by the patient's own pacemaker, whichever is the faster (Figure 38).

Other faults either in the pacemaker itself or in the pacing catheter may result in failure to pace (Figure 39). Permanent failure seldom happens

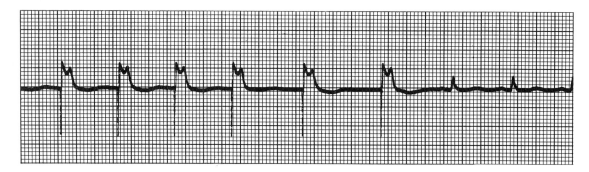

Figure 37. Pacemaker cutting out when patient's heart rate accelerates to 93 per minute.

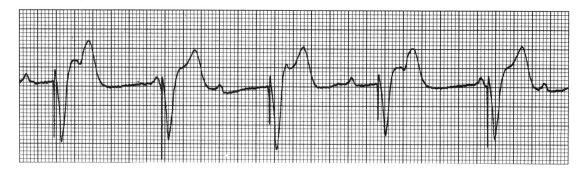

Figure 38. Failing battery pacing at 52 per minute.

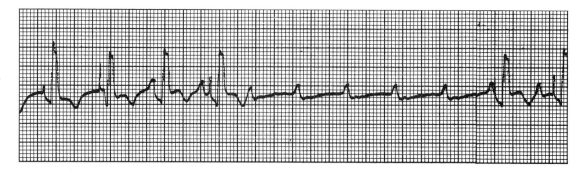

Figure 39. Fractured pacing wire within its sheath causing intermittent failure to pace.

nowadays without warning, but transient failure is not uncommon and the cause can be difficult to determine.

Patients who require pacemakers are in no way immune to other disorders of rate, rhythm and conduction, and these must be treated appropriately as and when they occur (Figure 40).

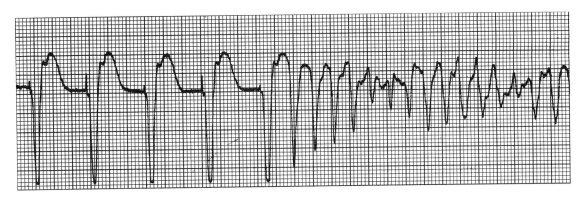

Figure 40. The onset of ventricular fibrillation in a paced patient.

Faulty Recordings

Badly fitted electrodes and loosely attached terminals cause many of the problems encountered when interpreting ECGs, especially in patients who are being continuously monitored with oscilloscopes or tape-recorders.

Under these circumstances, frequent shifting or distortion of the baseline not only makes interpretation difficult or impossible, but may also simulate serious abnormalities (Figures 41–45).

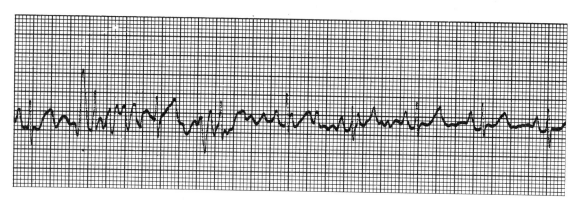

Figure 41. Record spoiled by baseline movement.

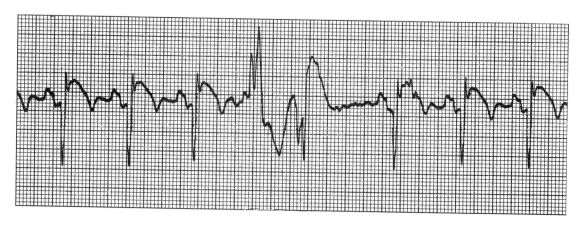

Figure 42. Patient movement simulating multifocal ventricular ectopic beats.

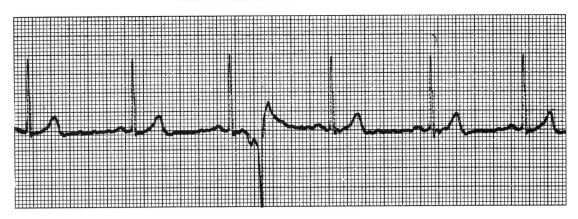

Figure 43. Patient movement simulating an R on T ventricular ectopic beat.

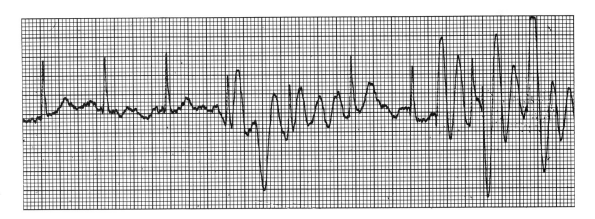

Figure 44. Badly fitted electrodes simulating ventricular fibrillation.

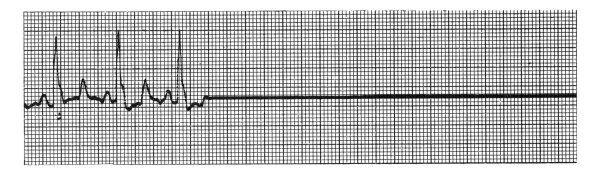

Figure 45. Loose terminal simulating asystolic arrest.

Some Sample Diagnoses

Example 1.

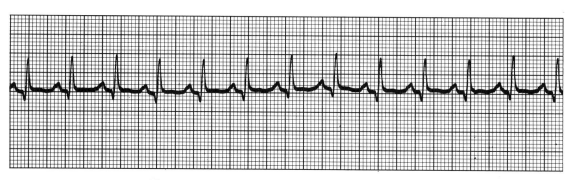

Figure 46.

In Figure 46:

- the P waves are readily identifiable
  - they are of normal width but of slightly bifid configuration
  - they occur at regular intervals
- the atrial rate is 124 per minute
- the QRS complexes are readily identifiable
  - they are of normal width and configuration
  - they occur at regular intervals
- the ventricular rate is 124 per minute
- the T waves are of very low voltage and difficult to identify
- there is one P wave for each QRS complex and they are constantly related to each other
- the PR interval is 0.16 seconds

Diagnosis: sinus tachycardia.

Example 2.

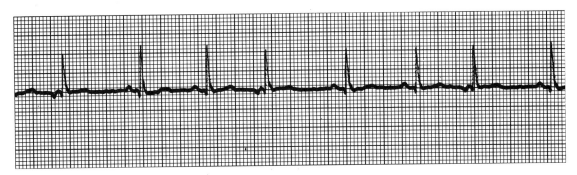

Figure 47.

In Figure 47:

- the P waves are readily identifiable
    - the 1st, 3rd, 4th, 6th and 7th are of normal width and configuration
    - the 2nd, 5th and 8th are of normal width and are inverted
    - the normal P waves occur at regular intervals but the abnormal P waves occur earlier than the next normal P would have been expected
    - each abnormal P wave is followed by a pause that is longer than the pause between two normal P waves (compensatory pauses)
    - following these pauses, the next normal P wave occurs when it would have been expected
- the atrial rate is 80 per minute
- the QRS complexes are readily identifiable
    - they are of normal width and configuration
    - they occur at the same regular intervals as the P waves
- the ventricular rate is 80 per minute
- the T waves are readily identifiable but are slightly flattened
- there is one P wave for each QRS complex
- the PR interval of the normal P waves is 0.14 seconds and of the inverted P waves is 0.10 seconds

Diagnosis: supraventricular ectopic beats (low atrial or possibly junctional in origin).

Example 3.

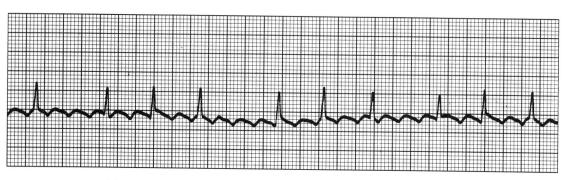

Figure 48.

In Figure 48:

- there are no normal P waves
- the QRS complexes are readily indentifiable
  - they are of normal width and configuration
  - they occur at irregular intervals
- the ventricular rate is approximately 100 per minute
- no T waves are visible
- the spaces between the QRS complexes are occupied by a continuum of regularly recurring saw-toothed deflections. These are abnormal P waves.
  - in some spaces there are 2 abnormal P waves
  - in some spaces there are 3 abnormal P waves
- the atrial rate is 280 per minute
- the P waves and the QRS complexes appear to be unrelated and there is no constant PR interval.

Diagnosis: atrial flutter.

Example 4.

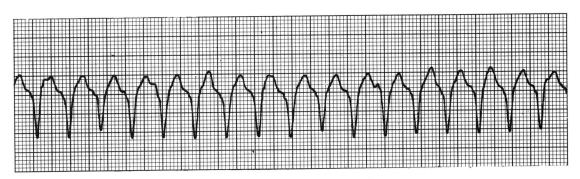

Figure 49.

In Figure 49:

- the P waves are not readily indentifiable
- the QRS complexes are readily indentifiable
  - they are broad and monophasic
  - they occur at regular intervals
- the ventricular rate is 175 per minute
- the T waves are readily identifiable
  - they point in the opposite direction to the QRS complexes
  - they are distorted here and there by deflections that might be P waves, but which have no constant relationship to the QRS complexes

Diagnosis: ventricular tachycardia.

Example 5.

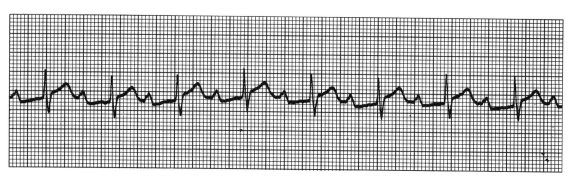

Figure 50.

In Figure 50:

- the P waves are readily indentifiable
  - they are of normal width and configuration
  - they occur at regular intervals
- the atrial rate is 80 per minute
- the QRS complexes are readily identifiable
  - they are of normal width and configuration
  - they occur at regular intervals
- the ventricular rate is 80 per minute
- the T waves are readily identifiable and of normal morphology
- there is one P wave for each QRS complex and they are constantly related to each other
- the PR interval is prolonged to 0.34 seconds

Diagnosis: sinus rhythm with 1st degree heart block.

Example 6.

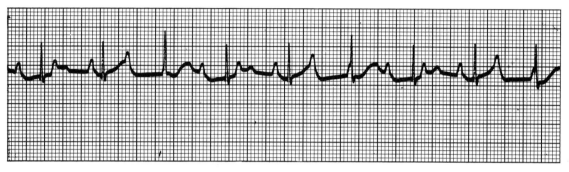

Figure 51.

In Figure 51:

- most of the P waves are readily identifiable
  - they are of normal width and configuration
  - they occur at regular intervals
  - some precede the QRS complexes
  - some are within the QRS complexes
  - some are in the ST-T wave segments
- the atrial rate is 150 per minute
- all the QRS complexes are readily identifiable
  - they are of normal width and configuration
  - they occur at regular intervals
- the ventricular rate is 86 per minute
- the T waves are distorted by P waves
- there are more P waves than QRS complexes and no relationship between them

Diagnosis: atrial tachycardia with atrioventricular dissociation.

Ladder diagrams

When analysis is difficult it is often helpful to construct a ladder diagram (Figure 52). The three rungs of the ladder represent:
- the atria
- the AV junctional tissues
- the ventricles

Vertical lines are drawn accurately under all the P waves to represent conduction through the atria. Vertical lines are drawn accurately under all the QRS complexes to represent conduction through the ventricles.

Only after this has been done should an attempt be made to join up the vertical lines through the AV rung of the ladder. It is sometimes also helpful to write the time intervals between the vertical lines.

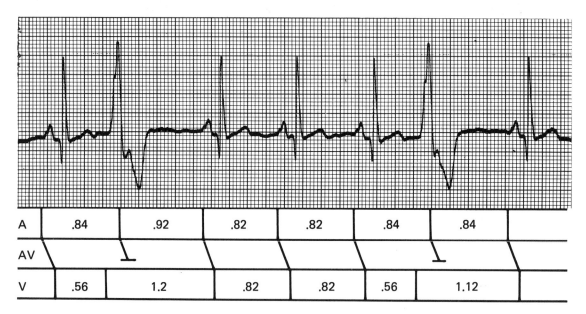

A	.84	.92	.82	.82	.84	.84	
AV							
V	.56	1.2	.82	.82	.56	1.12	

Figure 52. This is a ladder diagram showing two ventricular ectopic beats in a strip of sinus rhythm. They are easily recognised because the QRS complexes are broader that those of the normally conducted beats. Their morphology is also different, being initially positive instead of negative and they have a somewhat bizarre shape. Their T waves, as is customary, point in the opposite direction to the QRS complexes. Each is followed by a fully compensatory pause, i.e. the distance between the normal beats occurring before and after the ectopic beats is *twice* the distance between any two normal beats.

Despite the extrasystoles, the atrial rate remains constant throughout the record. The Ps can be easily identified on the downstroke of the ectopic T waves, but they are not followed by QRS complexes because the premature contractions have left the ventricles temporarily refractory to further stimulation.

32

2
PRESENTING FEATURES

Although disorders of rate, rhythm and conduction range from those that are of no consequence to those that are life-threatening, their importance, with a few notable exceptions, depends more on the state of the heart than upon the disorder itself. For example, whereas a rapid rate can be tolerated almost indefinitely by a healthy heart, tachycardia, by reducing the diastolic filling time, can soon cause symptoms in a heart that is already compromised by disease.

Even in the absence of a significant haemodynamic upset, patient response to disorders varies considerably. Some may be completely unaware of serious disturbances or have only modest symptoms, while others may become greatly alarmed if they become conscious of even relatively minor abnormalities.

Patients Without Symptoms

Many patients with disorders of rate, rhythm and conduction have no symptoms and are completely unaware of the abnormality. If it is drawn to their attention, the response varies. Some:
- remain unaware and unconcerned
- become aware but remain unconcerned
- become both aware and concerned

On the whole, it is best to say nothing about the discovery of such disorders to symptomless patients unless treatment is thought to be necessary.

Patients With Symptoms

In those who do have symptoms, the nature and severity of the symptoms may bear little or no relationship to the seriousness of the disorder. Some patients with potentially dangerous disorders of rate, rhythm and conduction have relatively few symptoms whilst others, who complain a lot, may be at little or no risk.

SYMPTOMS

Symptoms can be due either to awareness of the heart beat, often referred to as palpitation, or to the effects of disordered action of the heart on the efficiency of the cardiovascular system. The latter are more likely to occur if the heart is already diseased or malformed, and may result in:
- angina
- fatigue
- giddiness
- lightheadedness
- syncope
- heart failure

Awareness of the Heart Beat: Palpitation

It is not uncommon for healthy people to be aware of their heart beat. A few notice it during the night when lying quietly in bed, often on their left side. Many more become conscious of rapid beating in response to strenuous exertion or intense emotion.

Anxious patients are sometimes aware of sinus tachycardia and those with an increased cardiac output (e.g. severe aortic regurgitation, thyrotoxicosis) often notice the forceful contractions of their heart.

The nature of the palpitation and its cause can usually be determined by taking a proper history, carrying out a careful clinical examination and recording an ECG (sometimes it is necessary to use a 24-hour tape).

INVESTIGATION

Establish the complaint

When taking the history, it is extremely important to find out exactly what the patient is complaining about. In most cases, this will indicate that you are dealing with one or other of the following:
- normal cardiac action
- augmented cardiac action
- missed beats
- forceful beats
- rapid beats

Warning
The symptom known as **palpitation** means different things to different people and is sometimes difficult to interpret. Many patients are not familiar with the term.

If the answer to the question 'Do you ever have palpitation?' is 'No', *always* ask: 'Do you know what is meant by palpitation?' and surprisingly often the answer to this question is also 'No'.

DIAGNOSIS

If palpitation is caused by an abnormal reaction to normal circumstances, the way the story is told and the type of person telling it are usually fairly characteristic. If palpitation is the result of a hyperdynamic circulatory state, the associated clinical features usually make it fairly obvious that they are secondary to some other problem. *An important exception is masked thyrotoxicosis, a condition that is frequently missed in all types of practice.*

SYMPTOMS

Some patients give a clear description of missed or forceful beats, others refer to a strange feeling in the chest; but many are at a loss to find words to describe what they feel, and often place a hand over the upper precordium while trying to do so.

Careful questioning will reveal that the patient has become conscious of extra beats, the pause that follows them or, more often, the powerful contraction of the next normal beat, which has become augmented because of the prolonged diastolic filling time resulting from the pause. In these cases palpitation is due to ectopic beats (see pages 49, 67 and 73).

Patients with tachycardia usually describe rapid beating (thumping, fluttering, throbbing, pounding) over the precordium or sometimes in the root of the neck. This may be associated with a sensation of choking or feeling flushed.

Those who find it difficult to describe their symptoms are often helped to do so by being asked to tap out what they feel (i.e. the rate and rhythm) on the palm of the hand, the front of the sternum or the top of the table. Remember, however, that as the heart rate increases, it becomes progressively more difficult to count the rate accurately or to detect irregular spaces between beats without the help of an ECG.

After establishing that the patient has had tachycardia, the next thing to do is to determine whether it was constant or paroxysmal, and then whether it was regular or irregular.

If it was constant, the palpitation could have been due to one of the following:
- sinus tachycardia resulting from a wide variety of cardiac or non-cardiac causes (see page 44)
- atrial flutter (see page 62)
- atrial tachycardia, possibly due to intoxication with digitalis (see page 56)
- a prolonged attack of any of the paroxysmal tachycardias
  - either a first attack, or
  - the first attack of which the patient has become aware

If it was paroxysmal, determine whether it was occurring under circumstances where tachycardia might be expected, or if it was occurring for no apparent reason. If it was occurring for no apparent reason, you are probably dealing with paroxysmal tachycardia (see pages 52, 68 and 77).

To help assess the nature and severity of the attacks you should obtain the following information:
- how often the attacks occur
- how long they last
- has there been any change in their frequency or severity
- how an attack starts
- how an attack stops
- how fast the heart rate is during an attack

- whether the heart beats regularly or irregularly
- whether anything is known to precipitate an attack
- whether any way has been found to terminate an attack
- whether the attacks are accompanied by other symptoms such as
  - pain
  - breathlessness
  - giddiness
  - syncope

The answers to these questions should also help you to decide whether or not the attacks are frequent enough or troublesome enough to merit prophylactic or suppressive therapy.

Note. When you suspect that a patient has a disorder of rate, rhythm or conduction, always count both the pulse rate *and* the heart rate for at least 30 seconds and preferably for a full minute. This is because it is often helpful to know the exact rate from minute to minute. In sinus tachycardia, for example, it may vary slightly (138, 141, 139, 137), whereas in supraventricular tachycardia it will remain constant (138, 138, 138, 138). If the rate is counted for only 5 or 10 seconds and multiplied by 12 or 6, such important minor variations will not be apparent.

The Effects of Disordered Action of the Heart on the Efficiency of the Cardiovascular System

When the cardiovascular system is healthy, the heart rate has to be very fast or very slow to produce symptoms. But, when myocardial function is already poor or when the coronary, cerebral and other arteries are severely narrowed by atheroma, relatively minor disorders of rate, rhythm or conduction may cause significant deterioration in clinical status, and major disorders may rapidly become life-threatening. In these circumstances, any sudden or unexplained worsening of the patient's condition should immediately arouse suspicion that a disorder of rate, rhythm or conduction may be responsible, particularly in the elderly.

ASSOCIATED SYMPTOMS

Precordial pain or discomfort

Tachycardia, by increasing the demand of the myocardium for oxygen, frequently causes anginal pain in the presence of ischaemic heart disease. This sets up a vicious circle because the rapid rate has already reduced the cardiac output and the systemic blood pressure upon which the myocardium relies for an adequate blood supply.

If the heart rate is very fast and the attack is prolonged, it is not uncommon for the symptoms to mimic those of acute coronary insufficiency or even myocardial infarction. The myocardium may be permanently damaged if the tachycardia is not quickly controlled and the rate reduced to one that the already impaired coronary blood supply can sustain. In these circumstances, a correct diagnosis and adequate therapy are urgently required.

Anxious patients with sinus tachycardia often complain of precordial pain or discomfort. A careful history should differentiate this from genuine myocardial ischaemia.

Cerebral symptoms

Tachycardia or bradycardia may reduce cerebral blood flow below a critical level, especially if it is already compromised by cerebral vascular disease. Very rapid or very slow rates then produce symptoms varying in severity from giddiness or lightheadedness to mental confusion or even syncope. Many a patient is treated for epilepsy or ends up in a neurosurgical clinic whose slow pulse should have suggested that a cardiological opinion would have been more appropriate.

Heart failure

If patients whose cardiac reserves are low complain of increased breathlessness or fatigue, or if there is a sudden, unexplained deterioration in the cardiac status, a disorder of rate, rhythm or conduction should always be kept in mind as a possible cause of their symptoms.

3

VARIATIONS AND DISORDERS

Normal Sinus Rate and Rhythm

Before considering variations and disorders, let us look first at the normal case. In normal sinus rhythm, the rhythm is regular and the rate varies between 60 and 100 per minute (Figure 53). Anything less than 60 per minute is known as **sinus bradycardia**. Anything more than 100 per minute is known as **sinus tachycardia**. Neither is necessarily abnormal.

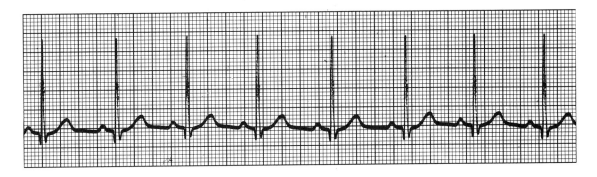

Figure 53. Normal sinus rhythm.

Variations Of Normal Heart Rates In Infants, Children And Adults

	Minimum	Mean	Maximum
Birth	95	125	165
1 week	100	140	190
1 month	110	150	200
3 months	115	150	180
6 months	110	135	160
1 year	95	120	150
3 years	90	100	125
5 years	70	95	115
10 years	65	80	110
15 years and over	60	72	100

VARIATIONS OF NORMAL SINUS RATE AND RHYTHM

The rate of impulse formation at the sinus node is constantly changing. It changes in response to *physiological* circumstances such as waking, sleeping or running and to *pathological* states such as anaemia, infections or heart failure. These changes are necessary to maintain an adequate circulation and most people are unaware that they are taking place.

Some normal people are aware of their heart beat, often when they are lying quietly in bed on the left side. In older patients, it is often a pulsation in the head or neck (frequently in the ear), rather than the heart itself, that reaches conscious level.

Many people notice an increase in heart rate during or after strenuous exercise or intense emotion and this is in no way abnormal. Anxious patients, too, are often conscious of what is going on in and around the precordium.

**VARIATIONS OF NORMAL
SINUS RATE AND RHYTHM**

- sinus bradycardia
- sinus tachycardia
- sinus dysrhythmia

Sinus Bradycardia

Sinus bradycardia is the term used to describe the heart rate in sinus rhythm if it is less than 60 per minute.

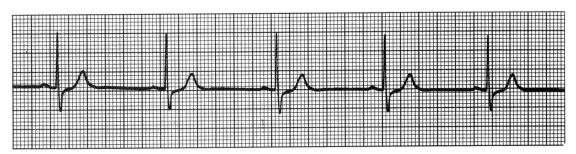

Figure 54. Sinus bradycardia.

Physiological bradycardia

Common in healthy people when they are at rest or asleep. It is especially noticeable in the young, in athletes and in the elderly, and is caused by increased vagal tone.

Pathological bradycardia

Causes
Convalescence from febrile illnesses, such as:
- influenza
- typhoid fever

Hypometabolic states, such as:
- hypothermia
- myxoedema

Diverse conditions, such as:
- vomiting
- obstructive jaundice
- raised intracranial pressure
- depressive psychoses
- early phase of myocardial infarction
- sick sinus syndrome
- tracheal intubation

41

Pharmacological bradycardia

Causes
Prescribed drugs, such as:
- beta blockers
- digitalis
- morphine
- reserpine

DIAGNOSIS

If the common causes are kept in mind there should be little or no doubt about the diagnosis.

Symptoms

There are usually no symptoms unless the ventricular rate is very slow in the presence of serious underlying heart disease.

Pulse and heart rate

The pulse and heart rates are slow, regular and equal. By definition, they are less than 60 per minute; in practice, seldom less than 45 per minute.

ECG

The ECG confirms the slow rate of less than 60 per minute. The P, QRS and T waves have a normal appearance and are normally related to each other (Figure 54).

Warning
Sinus bradycardia may be confused with more serious conditions. If the heart rate is totally irregular, the likely diagnosis is *atrial fibrillation with a slow ventricular rate.* If the heart is twice the slow pulse rate, the likely diagnosis is *coupled rhythm.* If the slow heart rate fails to increase in response to exercise, the likely diagnosis is *complete heart block* (see Figures 55–57).

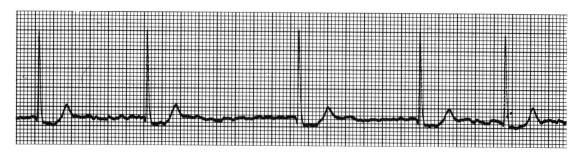

Figure 55. Atrial fibrillation with a slow ventricular rate.

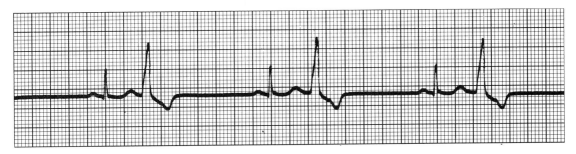

Figure 56. Coupled rhythm, pulse rate recorded as 34 per minute.

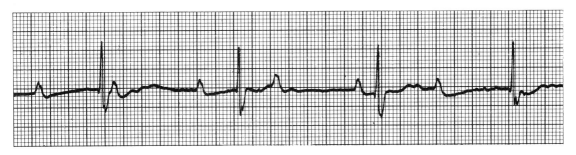

Figure 57. Complete heart block.

TREATMENT

Sinus bradycardia seldom requires treatment. A slow heart rate should be treated only when it gives rise to symptoms; never for its own sake.

If a patient is taking essential drugs known to cause bradycardia, the dose should not be reduced unless there is evidence of inadequate cardiac output and hypotension at rest or in response to exertion (fatigue, lightheadedness, syncope, etc.). This applies particularly to beta blockers.

If a patient is in the early phase of acute myocardial infarction (especially inferior infarction) treatment may be necessary to tide over a period of temporary instability. Initially, raise the foot of the bed, then give atropine sulphate 0.6 mg, and repeat after 10 and 30 minutes, if necessary.

If a patient has the sick sinus (tachycardia/bradycardia) syndrome, extreme bradycardia may cause Adams-Stokes-like symptoms and in these circumstances transvenous pacing is required.

Sinus Tachycardia

Sinus tachycardia is the term used to describe the heart rate in sinus rhythm if it is more than 100 per minute.

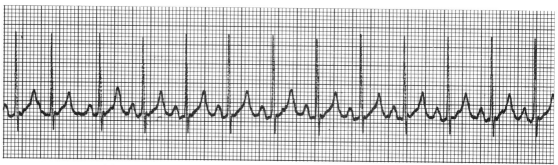

Figure 58. Sinus tachycardia.

Physiological tachycardia

Occurrence
In all healthy people during and after exercise, excitement, anxiety and other everyday emotions. In babies and infants the sinus rate is much faster. During childhood it gradually falls towards normal adult levels (see page 39).

Causes
Increased sympathetic activity or decreased vagal tone.

Pathological tachycardia

Causes
- fever
- anaemia
- hypoxia
- hypotension
- hyperthyroidism
- haemorrhage
- shock
- heart failure

Pharmacological tachycardia

Causes
- adrenaline
- ephedrine
- isoprenaline
- atropine
- alcohol
- nicotine
- caffeine

DIAGNOSIS

Symptoms

There are usually no symptoms. A few patients may complain of palpitation, but never of the sudden onset associated with paroxysmal tachycardia.

Pulse and heart rate

The pulse and heart rates are rapid, regular and equal. By definition they are more than 100 per minute; in practice, seldom more than 150 per minute. The maximum physiological response to exertion tends to decrease with age and poor physical condition.

ECG

The ECG confirms the rapid rate of more than 100 per minute. The P, QRS and T waves have a normal appearance and are normally related to each other (Figure 58).

Vagal stimulation
Carotid sinus massage, the valsalva manoeuvre or gagging may result in slight transient slowing of the heart rate, but usually has little or no effect.

Warning
Do not press on the patient's eyeballs; you may cause retinal damage and do more harm than good.

TREATMENT

Sinus tachycardia is nearly always a compensatory mechanism and does not require treatment. It should, however, direct attention to the *underlying cause*, which may or may not require treatment.

Sinus Dysrhythmia

Sinus dysrhythmia is the term used to describe variation in the sinus rate during the phases of respiration.

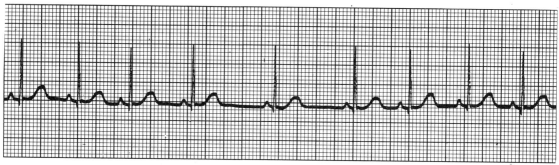

Figure 59. Sinus dysrhythmia.

AETIOLOGY

The heart rate accelerates during inspiration and slows during expiration.

Occurrence
Usually throughout the respiratory cycle.
Fairly obvious in children, young adults and the elderly.
Occasionally not obviously related to respiration.

Cause
Rhythmic fluctuations in vagal tone.

DIAGNOSIS

When pronounced, the irregular pulse may suggest other disorders of rhythm and conduction, but the diagnosis is seldom in doubt because the variation in the pulse and heart rate can nearly always be:
• exaggerated by increasing the depth and decreasing the rate of respiration
• abolished by increasing the heart rate

Symptoms

None.

46

Pulse and heart rate

The pulse and heart rates will be irregular if the variation is pronounced (see above). If it is not, the condition, which is of no consequence, is often an ECG diagnosis that is not noticed on clinical examination.

ECG

The ECG shows gradual lengthening and shortening of the distance between the QRS complexes, often referred to as the RR intervals. The P, QRS and T waves have a normal appearance and are normally related to each other unless another abnormality is also present (Figure 59).

TREATMENT

No treatment is necessary.

DISORDERS OF RATE, RHYTHM AND CONDUCTION

Rate, rhythm and conduction are in many ways interdependent. For example:
- a patient whose atria are fluttering 300 times per minute, but who has a 4:1 heart block, ends up with a normal ventricular (heart) rate of 75 despite the atrial tachycardia.
- a patient with a normal atrial rate of 75 and normal AV conduction, but who has ventricular tachycardia, ends up with a rapid ventricular (heart) rate of 160.
- a patient with an atrial tachycardia rate of 160, but who has a 2:1 heart block, ends up with a normal ventricular (heart) rate of 80.
- a patient with a normal atrial rate of 75, but who has complete heart block, ends up with a slow heart, because the idioventricular rate is only 50.

Remember that so far as the patient is concerned, it is the ventricular rate (heart rate) that matters and this must always be kept clearly in mind when considering management and treatment.

In practice, disorders of rate and rhythm are encountered much more frequently than disorders of conduction and, as they tend to be closely related, it is convenient to discuss them together before going on to consider disorders of conduction.

DISORDERS OF RATE AND RHYTHM

Disorders of Atrial Rate and Rhythm

- atrial ectopic beats
- supraventricular tachycardia
- atrial tachycardia with AV block
- atrial fibrillation
- atrial flutter

Disorders of Junctional (Nodal) Rate and Rhythm

- junctional (nodal) rhythm
- junctional (nodal) ectopic beats
- junctional (nodal) tachycardia
- wandering pacemaker
- reciprocal rhythms

Disorders of Ventricular Rate and Rhythm

- idioventricular rhythm
- ventricular ectopic beats
- ventricular tachycardia
- ventricular fibrillation
- ventricular standstill or asystole

DISORDERS OF CONDUCTION

- sinus block and arrest

- sick sinus (tachycardia/bradycardia) syndrome

Atrioventricular Block
- first degree AV block
- second degree AV block
  (Type I and Type II)
- bundle branch blocks
- third degree AV block
  (complete heart block)

- atrioventricular dissociation

- pre-excitation

DISORDERS OF ATRIAL RATE AND RHYTHM

Atrial Ectopic Beats

Atrial ectopic beats arise from sites in the atria other than the sinus node. They may be single or multiple. Although not necessarily premature or extra, the following terms are all used synonymously in clinical practice: ectopic beat, premature beat and extrasystole.

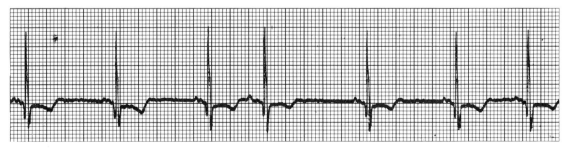

Figure 60. Atrial ectopic beat.

AETIOLOGY

Occurrence
- common in healthy people of all ages
- in patients with heart disease, they may predispose to or harbinger more serious atrial dysrhythmias

Precipitating factors
- emotional upset
- fatigue
- alcohol
- tobacco
- caffeine

Other causes
- atrial distension
- inflammation
- infiltration
- ischaemia

DIAGNOSIS

Symptoms

Atrial ectopic beats seldom cause symptoms. Some patients are conscious of missed beats or forceful contractions following compensatory pauses and complain of palpitation.

Pulse and heart rate

Single ectopic beats are felt or heard sooner than would be expected after a normal beat and are usually followed by a longer pause than would be expected between two normal beats.

Multiple ectopic beats result in an irregular pulse and heart and may be confused with atrial fibrillation. They always produce an audible first heart sound, but, if they occur too soon after the preceding beat, may not be palpable at the peripheral pulse.

ECG

The morphology of the P wave and its relationship to the QRS complex differs from those arising in the sinus node. The QRS complex is similar to the normal sinus beats and is usually followed by a compensatory pause (Figure 60). When there is no compensatory pause, the ectopic beat is said to be **interpolated**.

Caution
Difficulties in the interpretation of the ECG may arise if:
- the premature P wave occurs on the T wave of the preceding normal beat (Figure 61)

- there is aberrant conduction of the premature atrial impulse down the left or right bundle branches, with the result that the QRS complex resembles a ventricular ectopic beat (Figure 62)
- the premature atrial impulse arrives at the AV node while the junctional tissues are still refractory, in which case the abnormal P wave is not followed by a QRS complex (Figure 63)

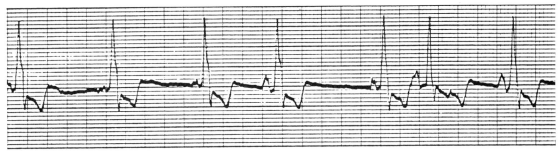

Figure 61. Premature P on preceding T.

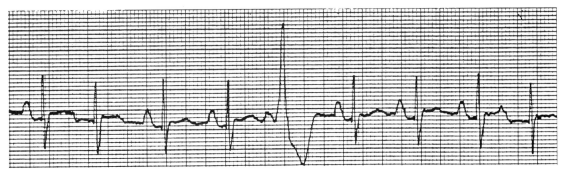

Figure 62. Aberrant conduction resembling ventricular ectopic beat.

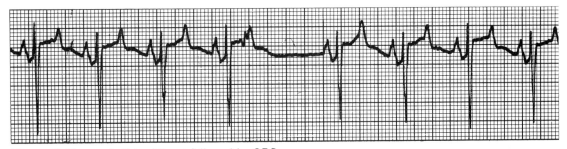

Figure 63. Very early P (on T) not followed by QRS.

TREATMENT

Atrial ectopic beats seldom require treatment. It is worthwhile searching for a possible cause, but in practice it is seldom rewarding. If symptoms remain troublesome, even after reassurance, they can usually be suppressed with digoxin or a beta blocker.

51

Supraventricular Tachycardia

Theoretically, the term applies to all tachycardias that arise above the bifurcation of the His bundle, because the AV node and bundle lie in the lower part of the right atrium. Although this definition should include sinus tachycardia, atrial flutter and atrial fibrillation, in practice, it usually refers to paroxysms of atrial or junctional tachycardia.

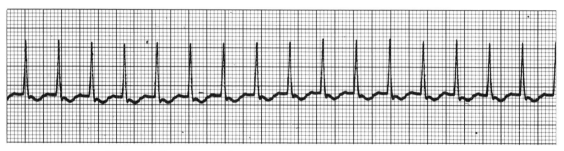

Figure 64. Supraventricular tachycardia.

AETIOLOGY

Occurrence
This is the commonest type of paroxysmal tachycardia at all ages in those with normal and abnormal hearts. Most younger patients appear in all other respects healthy.

Others may have:
- rheumatism
- coronary, pulmonary or thyroid heart disease
- a prolapsed mitral valve cusp
- Wolff-Parkinson-White syndrome
- Lown-Ganong-Levine syndrome
- sick sinus syndrome

Precipitating factors
Tea, coffee, tobacco, alcohol, exercise, emotional upset.

Note. As a rule, there is no obvious reason why an ectopic focus assumes enhanced automaticity or a circuit of re-entry becomes established.

DIAGNOSIS

Characteristically, the attack starts suddenly and the patient is immediately aware of the change. Sometimes it also ends suddenly, although the rate often slows gradually; the attack tails off and the patient is unaware of the change first to sinus tachycardia and then to normal sinus rhythm.

The length of attacks may vary from a few moments to hours or even days, but they are usually fairly short-lived.

SYMPTOMS

Some patients are unaware of attacks. Some notice fluttering or pounding in the chest or neck. Some have symptoms such precordial pain, breathlessness or a choking feeling in the throat.

The rate is important. Slower rates are tolerated better and longer than faster ones. A very rapid heart rate may soon cause weakness, fatigue and lightheadedness.

Pulse and heart rate

The pulse and heart rates are rapid, regular and equal. The rate may vary within wide limits (100–300), but is usually between 140 and 220 per minute and frequently in the region of 160–180. Vagal stimulation either terminates the paroxysm or has no effect upon it.

With very rapid rates it is often difficult, on clinical examination, to appreciate minor irregularities between beats, as in atrial fibrillation with a fast ventricular rate. There is never any doubt about it, however, when the peaks of the R waves are plotted out on an ECG.

ECG

Normal QRS complexes occur rapidly and with absolute regularity. P waves may or may not be present. Each QRS complex is constantly related to an abnormal P wave, if P waves are present (Figure 64).

As the rate increases it becomes increasingly difficult to disentangle the P waves from the preceding T waves. If the right or left bundle branch is refractory to the rapid propagation of impulses, aberrant conduction causes wide QRS complexes that give a false impression of ventricular tachycardia, and it may be difficult or impossible to differentiate between them on a single record (Figures 65–67).

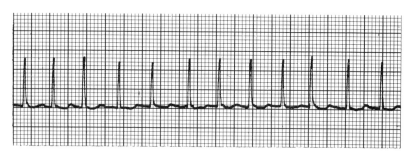

Figure 65. Atrial fibrillation with a fast ventricular rate.

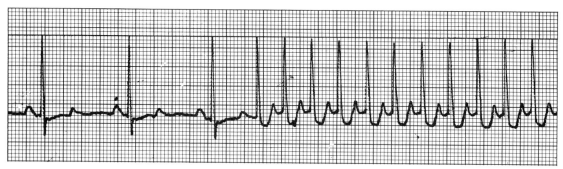

Figure 66. Supraventricular tachycardia with normal conduction.

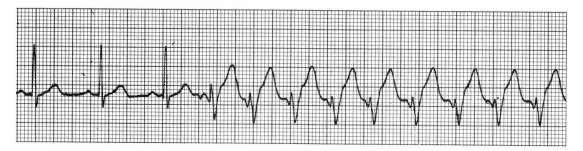

Figure 67. Supraventricular tachycardia with aberrant conduction.

TREATMENT

The need for treatment depends upon the length and frequency of attacks, the heart rate during attacks and the patient's reaction to them. Many attacks are self-terminating, with a spontaneous return to sinus rhythm (Figure 68). Most patients would see little point in taking daily prophylaxis to prevent a ten-minute paroxysm once or twice a month.

54

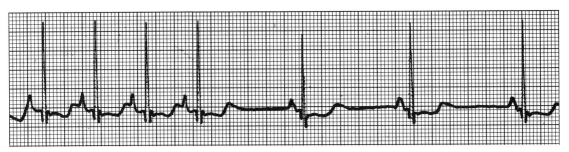

Figure 68. Spontaneous return to sinus rhythm.

Precipitating factors should be sought for and eliminated if possible. As a rule, none is discovered. Reassurance is all that is needed in many cases; sometimes reinforced with mild sedation.

If vagal stimulation is effective in terminating attacks (see page 154), patients should be taught to do this, for example, by gagging or performing a Valsalva manoeuvre. If they are unable to do this, or if it is ineffective, they should lie down quietly in a darkened room holding deep breaths for as long as possible, until the paroxysm stops or wears off.

If suppressive therapy is required, give digoxin. If this is ineffective, try a beta blocker. When paroxysms are difficult to control, verapamil, disopyramide, quinidine or amiodarone can be used. (See 'Treatment', pages 156, 134, 150, 122).

If the rapid rate is causing serious haemodynamic consequences in patients with underlying heart disease, intravenous therapy or cardioversion with a DC shock may be necessary.

Caution

If a combination of drugs is required, remember that verapamil when given with a beta blocker has powerful negative inotropic effects and in *fully digitalised* patients may cause asystole.

Atrial Tachycardia with AV Block

This type of atrial tachycardia resembles supraventricular tachycardia in that an ectopic focus or re-entry circuit causes the atria to contract rapidly at a rate of between 140 and 220 per minute, but differs from it by being accompanied by a variable degree of AV block (often 2:1) (Figure 69). Although customarily referred to as **paroxysmal atrial tachycardia with block**, it is not a truly paroxysmal disorder.

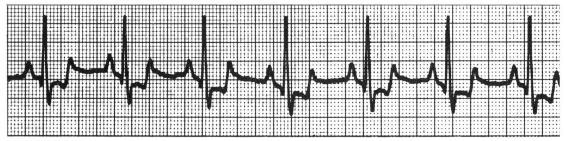

Figure 69. Paroxysmal atrial tachycardia with 2:1 AV block.

AETIOLOGY

Atrial tachycardia with AV block is frequently associated with serious heart disease.

Occurrence
It is much less common than paroxysmal supraventricular tachycardia. It should always be kept in mind as a possible reason for clinical deterioration in patients who are already ill with serious organic heart disease.

Especially
• in those undergoing intensive medical treatment
• in elderly patients on full adult doses of digoxin

Cause
Frequently a manifestation of digitalis toxicity.

Precipitating factors
Sometimes by depletion of cellular potassium due to:
• diarrhoea
• vomiting
• powerful potassium-losing diuretics

DIAGNOSIS

This potentially serious disorder cannot be diagnosed at the bedside. It is usually unsuspected or mistaken for some other abnormality.

The clinical features depend upon the atrial rate and the degree of AV block. With rapid rates (140–220 per minute), the AV node may be unable to conduct every impulse and the ventricles often respond only to alternate atrial beats. Too much digitalis increases the degree of block.

Symptoms

These depend upon the ventricular rate and the state of the myocardium. They vary from none, to those suggesting heart failure.

Pulse and heart rate

In severe heart block, the ventricular rate is usually between 70 and 110 per minute, and in these circumstances the pulse and heart rate suggest either normal sinus rhythm or sinus tachycardia.

If the block is less severe, the passage of atrial impulses is delayed rather than blocked, the ventricles respond to each beat and the rate is between 140 and 220 per minute.

If the heart block is variable, the pulse and heart rates are irregular and the condition may be mistaken for atrial fibrillation.

ECG

An ECG is essential for diagnosis.

The QRS complexes are of normal configuration, but the P waves differ from those in sinus rhythm and may be:
- small and narrow
- tall and spiked

The PR interval of conducted beats is:
- prolonged in first degree block
- normal in 2:1 block, where two P waves are seen between each QRS complex

Atrial tachycardia with block is easily distinguished from atrial flutter by:
- the slower atrial rate (140–220 compared with 280–320)
- the iso-electric line between P waves gives an even base-line rather than the continuous saw-toothed appearance common in flutter.

Vagal stimulation sometimes produces a response like that seen in atrial flutter, but quite unlike that seen in paroxysmal supraventricular tachycardia. By increasing the degree of AV block, it may cause transient slowing of the ventricular rate without influencing the atrial tachycardia.

TREATMENT

Patients who are taking digitalis should be treated as cases of digitalis toxicity until proved otherwise – i.e:

- stop digitalis therapy
- give a potassium supplement
- prescribe a beta blocker if the ventricular rate is rapid

If haemodynamic deterioration has occurred and treatment is urgently required, IV phenytoin should be used in preference to a DC shock.

Patients who have *not* had digitalis require no treatment unless the ventricular rate is very fast. In these circumstances it can usually be slowed by giving digoxin. Sometimes it is necessary to add a beta blocker if digoxin alone is inadequate. Occasionally, in an emergency, a DC shock is required.

Atrial Fibrillation

Purposeful atrial contraction is replaced by ineffective writhing of the atrial myocardium, hence the analogy to a bag of worms. A multitude of rapidly recurring stimuli of varying intensity constantly bombard the AV node, which is refractory to most of them. Those that are conducted are conducted randomly, and this results in a totally irregular ventricular rate (Figure 70).

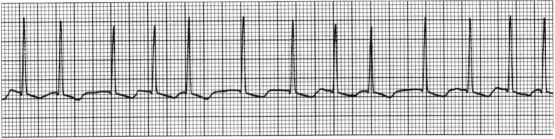

Figure 70. Atrial fibrillation.

AETIOLOGY

Occurrence
Atrial fibrillation is most commonly seen as a late complication:
- of rheumatic, ischaemic, hypertensive or thyroid heart disease
- in serious conditions involving the atrial walls (often infiltrative)
- when the atria become dilated as a result of increased pressure

Less commonly
- as lone atrial fibrillation in apparently healthy adults
- in diseases involving other systems (particularly the lungs)

Cause – uncertain, but possibly
- multiple areas of enhanced automaticity
- re-entry circuits
- both

DIAGNOSIS

Atrial fibrillation is much commoner than any of the other significant supraventricular dysrhythmias. It is the commonest cause of a pulse that is totally irregular in both time and force.

Multiple ectopic beats are sometimes confused with it, but occasional periods of regular rhythm nearly always provide a clue to the correct diagnosis.

When the ventricular rate is very rapid, the irregularity in time between contractions is clinically less obvious, although the irregularity in their force remains. This is manifest by:

- the varying intensity of the first heart sound
- the detection of a pulse deficit (more first heart sounds are heard than radial pulses are felt)

When the ventricular rate is slow, either naturally or under the influence of digitalis, the clinical diagnosis is much more difficult and can often be confirmed only with the help of an ECG (Figure 71).

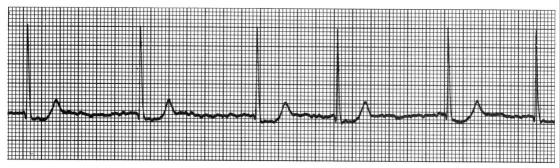

Figure 71. Atrial fibrillation (ventricular rate slowed by digoxin).

Atrial fibrillation sometimes occurs in paroxysms before becoming the established rhythm. In these circumstances patients are sometimes aware of palpitation or conscious of the change from one rhythm to the other.

SYMPTOMS

Some patients have no symptoms related to their atrial fibrillation and are unaware of it. Some have palpitation or are conscious of an irregular heart beat when it speeds up in response to exertion or excitement.

Some have symptoms that are dictated by the ventricular rate and the state of the myocardium. These vary from gradual deterioration of effort tolerance to sudden heart failure. Heart failure occurs when cardiac output falls below a critical level as a result of reduced diastolic filling time and loss of atrial transport function because the atria no longer contract.

Atrial stasis may lead to thrombosis, especially in mitral stenosis, and this predisposes to peripheral and pulmonary embolism in patients who are not on anticoagulant therapy.

Pulse and heart rate

The pulse and heart beats are irregular in time and force. The ventricular rate is usually between 100 and 150 per minute, but may be more or less. A pulse deficit occurs when the heart rate is rapid, because many of the ineffective beats do not produce a peripheral pulse.

ECG

The ECG shows absence of P waves, normal QRS complexes and totally irregular RR intervals. The chaotic atrial activity is manifest by irregular undulation of the iso-electric line between the ventricular potentials. Often they are barely visible, but sometimes they are large enough to be mistaken for P waves or flutter waves (particularly in V_1). The variation in their size and shape, plus the absence of a fixed relationship to the QRS complexes, should prevent confusion.

TREATMENT

Patients with serious heart disease should have a rapid ventricular rate slowed as quickly as possible with digoxin. In emergencies the first dose can be given intravenously. Sometimes a beta blocker is also required to achieve adequate control.

After the ventricular rate is controlled, a decision must be made about whether or not to attempt to restore sinus rhythm by DC cardioversion. This is usually not advised if the fibrillation has occurred in the natural course of a chronic disease, unless it has been precipitated prematurely.

Cardioversion is helpful in acute myocardial infarction, pneumonia and thyrotoxicosis, if the rapid ventricular rate is causing haemodynamic upset, or does not revert spontaneously with treatment of the underlying disease. It is seldom successful in lone atrial fibrillation.

Atrial Flutter

In this type of atrial tachycardia, the atria contract regularly about 300 times per minute. The AV node can rarely conduct so many rapidly recurring impulses and is usually refractory to at least half of them.

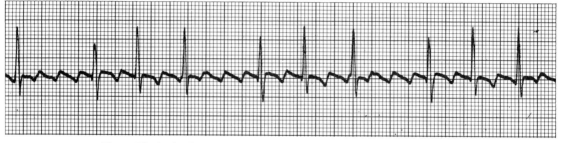

Figure 72. Atrial flutter with AV block varying from 2:1 to 4:1.

AETIOLOGY

Atrial flutter is uncommon in the absence of heart disease. It may complicate rheumatic, ischaemic or thyroid heart disease, myocarditis or cardiomyopathies.

Occurrence
- usually in already diseased hearts
- sometimes paroxysmal, but more commonly an established rhythm

Cause
- probably an atrial ectopic pacemaker firing off at a very rapid rate, possibly with the assistance of a re-entry circuit. The theory of circus rhythm is currently out of favour.

DIAGNOSIS

Although the atrial rate is usually between 280 and 320 per minute, the clinical features depend upon the ventricular rate, which in turn depends upon the degree of block in the AV junctional tissues. Very occasionally all the atrial impulses are conducted to the ventricle (1:1 flutter) and few, even healthy hearts, can tolerate the resulting ventricular rate of around 300 per minute for long without failing.

Symptoms

There are usually no symptoms unless the ventricular rate is very rapid and the patient has serious underlying heart disease. Some patients are conscious of a change in heart rate if the degree of heart block is unstable.

Pulse and heart rate

The pulse and heart rates are usually regular and equal. If the AV block is variable, the rate will be irregular and abrupt changes may be noted.

With 2:1 block, the rate is 140–160 per minute.
With 3:1 block, the rate is 95–110 per minute.
With 4:1 block, the rate is 70–80 per minute.

ECG

The ECG shows a typical saw-toothed pattern with no iso-electric line between regularly recurring P waves (Figure 72).

In 2:1 block, the apex of every second P may be lost in the preceding QRS complex (Figure 73). It is revealed when the degree of block changes either spontaneously or as a result of vagal stimulation. When the degree of block changes, the ventricular rates have a common denominator. Sometimes the PR interval is constant; sometimes it is not.

These features of atrial flutter are not always obvious in all leads. They are best seen in leads 2, 3, aVF or V_1.

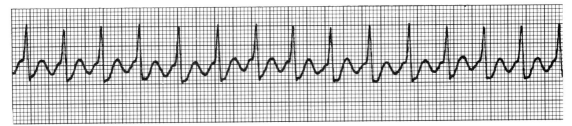

Figure 73. 2:1 atrial flutter.

Aid to diagnosis
Vagal stimulation often induces a transient increase in the degree of AV block and helps to reveal the true nature of the tachycardia (Figure 74).

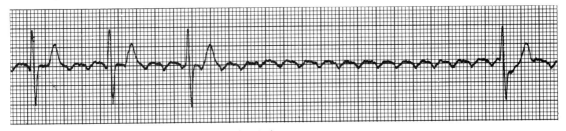

Figure 74. Atrial flutter – response to vagal stimulation.

63

TREATMENT

The treatment of choice is to cardiovert with a DC shock. As a rule, only a small electrical charge (25–50 Ws) is required to restore normal rhythm (Fig. 75).

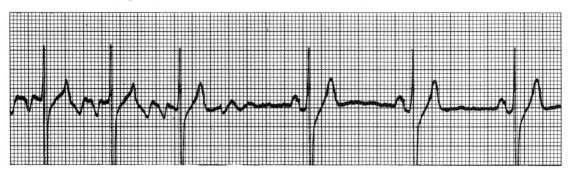

Figure 75. Atrial flutter – change to sinus rhythm following cardioversion.

The drug of choice is probably still digoxin. It acts by increasing the degree of AV block and keeps the ventricular rate under control. Patients whose flutter is likely to recur should be kept on a maintenance dose. Other drugs, such as beta blockers, quinidine and disopyramide, may be used with varying degrees of success.

Important
Quinidine should never be given without digoxin – *given alone it may facilitate 1:1 conduction.*

DISORDERS OF JUNCTIONAL (NODAL) RATE AND RHYTHM

Until fairly recently it was thought that the AV node itself was the junctional pacemaker. It is now known that the His bundle is also involved and the term **junctional** is used with increasing frequency to designate rhythms that are neither atrial nor ventricular in origin.

The AV junction becomes the site of impulse formation if:
- the sinus pacemaker fails
- the automaticity of the sinus pacemaker falls below that of a junctional pacemaker
- the automaticity of a junctional pacemaker rises above that of the sinus pacemaker

When a junctional pacemaker takes over, the impulse is conducted forwards and downwards to the ventricles (antegrade conduction), and backwards and upwards to the atria (retrograde conduction).

Junctional Rhythm

Junctional (nodal) rhythm is said to exist when a site in the AV junctional tissues has taken over the pacemaker function of the heart. It is often still referred to as nodal rhythm. When due to failure of the sinus node, the rate is usually between 50 and 60 per minute. When due to enhanced automaticity of a junctional pacemaker, the rate is usually between 60 and 100 per minute, and this is known as accelerated junctional rhythm.

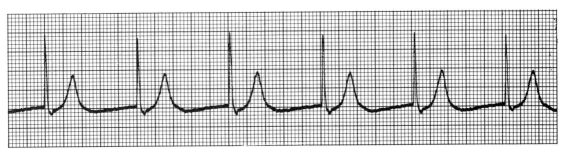

Figure 76. Junctional rhythm.

65

AETIOLOGY

Anything that suppresses sinus node activity or enhances AV junctional activity may result in a junctional rhythm.

Causes
- increased vagal tone
- digitalis
- rheumatic fever
- myocarditis
- myocardial infarction

Frequently no cause is apparent.

DIAGNOSIS

The condition is usually unsuspected.

Symptoms

None.

Pulse and heart rate

The pulse and heart rate are usually normal and equal, but may be either abnormally fast or slow.

ECG

Junctional rhythm is an ECG diagnosis. The QRS complexes appear to be normal (Figure 76), but the P waves may precede, coincide with or follow them depending upon the site of the pacemaker within the junctional tissues and the speed of conduction through them. Sometimes there are no P waves. When present, they are inverted in lead 2.

TREATMENT

As a rule, none is required.

Junctional Ectopic Beats

Junctional (nodal) ectopic beats are similar to atrial ectopic beats.

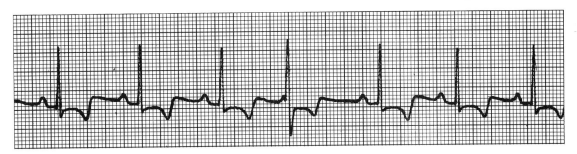

Figure 77. Junctional ectopic beat.

DIAGNOSIS

They can be differentiated from atrial ectopic beats only with the help of an ECG, if the record shows P waves occurring immediately before, within (Figure 77) or immediately after the QRS complexes.

TREATMENT

Like atrial ectopic beats, junctional beats are of little or no consequence and seldom require treatment.

Junctional Tachycardia

Junctional (nodal) tachycardia is the term used when the heart rate is more than 100 per minute and the pacemaker is in the junctional tissues.

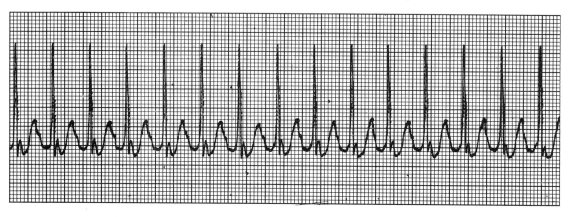

Figure 78. Junctional tachycardia.

DIAGNOSIS

Junctional tachycardia is similar in many ways to supraventricular tachycardia (see page 52). It can only be diagnosed electrocardiographically, the P waves and their relationship to the QRS complexes providing the clue, if they can be identified (Figure 78).

TREATMENT

As for supraventricular tachycardia.

Wandering Pacemaker

This is the term used when the pacemaker shifts backwards and forwards from the SA node to the junctional tissues or other foci in the atria.

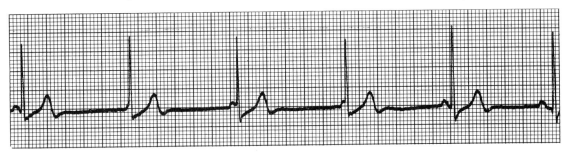

Figure 79. Wandering pacemaker.

AETIOLOGY

It may appear in normal hearts, where it is probably due to fluctuating vagal tone. It is also seen in various types of heart disease, notably in acute rheumatism and in patients receiving digitalis.

DIAGNOSIS

ECG

The ECG shows normal QRS complexes with P waves that differ in size, shape and polarity. Their relationship to the QRS complexes varies and some may be buried within them (Figure 79).

TREATMENT

None is required.

Reciprocal Rhythm

When an impulse arises in the junctional tissues or the ventricles, it travels forwards to activate the ventricles and backwards to activate the atria. If it then travels back down again to activate the ventricles for a second time, this second beat is known as a **reciprocal** or **echo beat**.

An impulse circulating round in the junctional tissues may produce a reciprocating tachycardia.

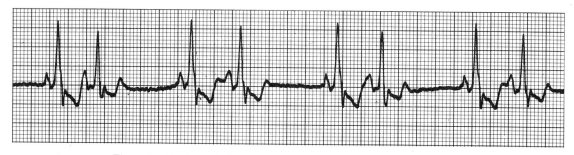

Figure 80. Reciprocal rhythm.

AETIOLOGY

Reciprocal rhythms are usually due either to some primary disturbance such as myocardial ischaemia or to the pharmacological action of drugs such as digitalis.

DIAGNOSIS

A reciprocal beat is a special kind of ectopic beat and can only be diagnosed with the help of an ECG. It should be suspected if a P wave is seen to separate two identical or nearly identical QRS complexes that occur closer together than would normally be expected (Figure 80).

TREATMENT

No treatment is required for reciprocal beats. Reciprocal tachycardia is treated as supraventricular tachycardia.

DISORDERS OF VENTRICULAR RATE AND RHYTHM

Idioventricular Rhythm

This is a condition in which the ventricles function independently of the atria or junctional tissues under the control of an ectopic ventricular pacemaker.

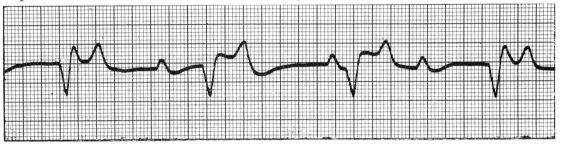

Figure 81. Idioventricular rhythm.

AETIOLOGY

Occurrence
When supraventricular impulses are absent or are not conducted through the AV junctional tissues and the AV junctional tissues do not take over the pacemaker function of the heart.

Cause
Usually a manifestation of complete heart block.

DIAGNOSIS

Symptoms

There may be symptoms suggesting low cardiac output when the ventricular rate is very slow.

Pulse and heart rate

The pulse and heart rate are slow, regular and equal: often between 20 and 40 per minute. The rate responds only slightly or not at all to circumstances that normally cause it to accelerate, such as emotion, exertion etc.

ECG

The ECG shows broad QRS complexes occurring regularly at a slow rate. Regularly recurring P waves are usually present also, but they occur at two or three times the ventricular rate and bear no relationship to the QRS complexes (Figure 81).

Accelerated idioventricular rhythm

When the heart rate is more than 40–50 but less than 100 per minute, the term accelerated idioventricular rhythm is used (Figure 82). This is preferred to 'slow ventricular tachycardia', because it is most often seen following acute myocardial infarction, where the term ventricular tachycardia has a completely different connotation.

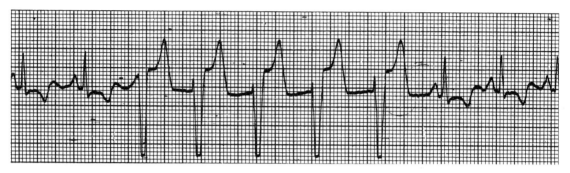

Figure 82. Short run of accelerated idioventricular rhythm.

TREATMENT

The need for treatment depends upon the nature of the condition causing the underlying complete heart block (see page 99).

Ventricular Ectopic Beats

Ventricular ectopic beats can arise from an ectopic focus anywhere in either ventricle. They may be single or multiple, and although not necessarily either premature or extra, the terms ectopic beat, premature beat and extrasystole are all used synonymously in clinical practice.

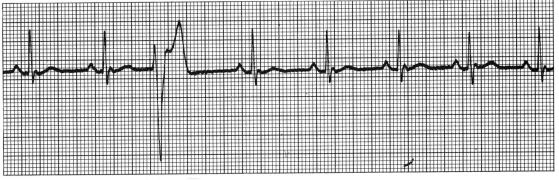

Figure 83. Ventricular ectopic beats.

AETIOLOGY

Occurrence
Ventricular ectopic beats are not uncommon in apparently healthy people and are of no significance. They are also common in patients with organic heart disease, particularly if the myocardium is affected by:
- coronary heart disease
- cardiomyopathies

Causes
An ectopic focus in the ventricles may initiate ectopic beats by:
- enhanced automaticity
- a re-entry circuit
- ventricular escape, if the sinus node and the junctional pacemakers are suppressed

Precipitating factors
- increased vagal tone
- emotional upset
- fatigue
- caffeine
- alcohol
- tobacco
- sympathomimetic drugs

Other causes

Too much digitalis is a common cause in patients with heart disease on long-term treatment, especially when diuretic therapy has caused potassium depletion. Coupled rhythm (an ectopic beat following each normal beat) is often due to digitalis intoxication (Figure 84).

Figure 84. Coupled rhythm.

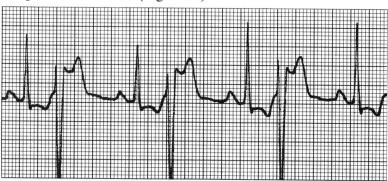

DIAGNOSIS

Most people are unaware of ectopic beats, and they seldom give rise to symptoms.

Symptoms

Some patients are conscious of missed beats or extra forceful beats following compensatory pauses, especially if they are numerous and occur frequently.

Pulse and heart rate

Single ectopic beats are felt or heard sooner than would be expected after a normal beat, and are usually followed by a longer pause than would be expected between two normal beats. Multiple ectopic beats result in an irregular pulse and heart rate, and may be confused with atrial fibrillation. They always produce an audible first heart sound, but, if they occur too soon after the preceding beat, may not be palpable at the peripheral pulse.

ECG

The ECG shows wide, bizarre QRS complexes with T waves pointing in the opposite direction. This abnormal ventricular complex is not preceded by a P wave, although P waves can often be seen distorting the QRS or T deflections (Figure 83).

An ectopic beat is usually followed by a compensatory pause; if not, it is referred to as being 'interpolated' (Figures 85 and 86).

When caused by an ectopic focus or by re-entry, it usually occurs soon after the previous normal complex. If it is an escape mechanism, it usually occurs later.

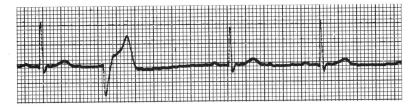

Figure 85. Ectopic beat followed by a compensatory pause.

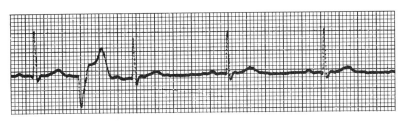

Figure 86. Interpolated ectopic beat.

Ectopic beats with the same morphology are assumed to arise from the same site in the ventricular myocardium. When their morphology differs, they are said to be 'multifocal' (Figure 87). When they point in opposite directions they are said to be 'bidirectional' (Figure 88).

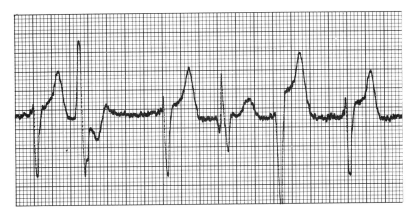

Figure 87. Multifocal ectopic beats.

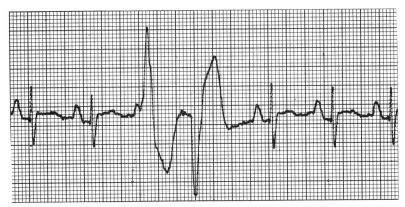

Figure 88. Bidirectional ectopic beats.

TREATMENT

- in most cases ventricular ectopic beats do not require treatment
- possible causes, particularly overdosage with digitalis or diuretics should be corrected
- ectopic beats that are troublesome can be suppressed
- following myocardial infarction, certain types of ventricular ectopic beats (R on T) may initiate ventricular tachycardia or ventricular fibrillation and call for prophylactic therapy (Figure 89)

Figure 89. R on T ectopic beat.

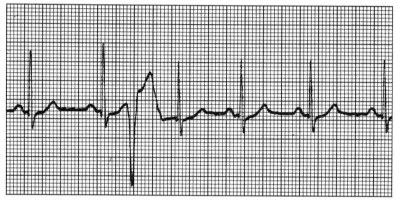

The choice of drugs would include:
- lignocaine
- tocainide
- mexilitine
- disopyramide
- sotalol

Ventricular Tachycardia

In theory two or more consecutive ventricular ectopic beats at a rate equivalent to more than 100 per minute constitute a run of ventricular tachycardia (VT). In practice, many more are required and at a much faster rate before this abnormal rhythm assumes clinical significance. A decision about how many consecutive beats constitute tachycardia is arbitrary and varies from centre to centre. A typical scheme might be for less than nine to be regarded as a run of ventricular ectopic beats, and more than nine as ventricular tachycardia.

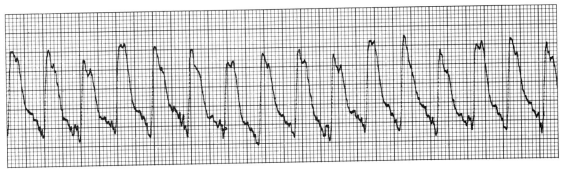

Figure 90. Ventricular tachycardia.

AETIOLOGY

Occurrence
Ventricular tachycardia is a serious complication of severe organic heart disease. It *occasionally* occurs in apparently healthy patients.

Causes
- myocardial ischaemia or infarction
- numerous drugs, of which digitalis is the most common offender

DIAGNOSIS

Attacks occur in paroxysms lasting from a few seconds to many hours.

Symptoms

Palpitation may be the first symptom, but if the rate is rapid and the myocardium diseased, this is rapidly followed by breathlessness, anginal pain, hypotension, shock and acute heart failure.

Pulse and heart rate

The pulse and heart rates are rapid, regular and equal. The rate is usually between 140 and 220 per minute. It does not respond to vagal stimulation.

ECG

The ECG shows a succession of rapidly recurring ventricular ectopic beats which are often slightly irregular (Figures 90 and 91). In most cases there is AV dissociation, and the P waves are usually difficult to see except as occasional notches or irregularities occurring inconsistently throughout the record. In a few cases, there is retrograde conduction to the atria, and P waves may be seen following the bizarre QRS complexes. As the rate increases, it becomes increasingly difficult to separate the broad QRS complexes from their ST-T wave segments, and the tracing gives the impression of a series of large, wide undulations with little or no iso-electric line between them (Figure 92). Sometimes the ventricular tachycardia changes almost imperceptibly into ventricular fibrillation.

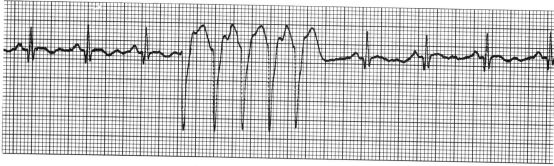

Figure 91. Short run of consecutive ventricular ectopic beats.

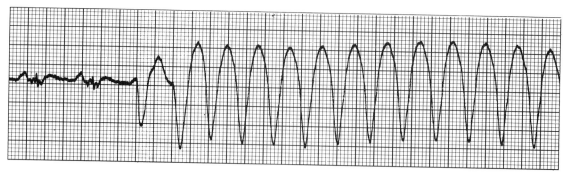

Figure 92. Undulating ventricular tachycardia.

When one of the bundle branches is refractory, it can be very difficult or sometimes impossible with ordinary ECG leads to differentiate between ventricular tachycardia (VT) and supraventricular tachycardia (SVT) with aberration (Figure 93). The following points are sometimes helpful:
- both may be regular, but slight irregularity favours VT
- vagal stimulation may terminate SVT, but has no effect on VT
- a QRS pattern suggesting right bundle branch block in V_1 favours SVT
- at the start of the paroxysm, an abnormal P wave, often superimposed on the preceding T wave, favours SVT
- P wave evidence of AV dissociation is diagnostic of VT

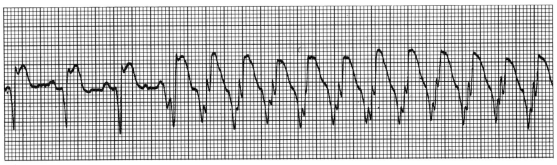

Figure 93. Supraventricular tachycardia with aberration.

TREATMENT

Immediate action is called for, especially following recent myocardial infarction, when ventricular tachycardia is a frequent precursor of ventricular fibrillation, the commonest cause of death during the early phase of the acute illness.

If the patient's condition is good, initiate treatment with one of the following:
- lignocaine
- disopyramide
- mexiletine

Move on to oral:
- disopyramide
- mexiletine
- quinidine
- procainamide
- tocainide
- sotalol

If rapid haemodynamic deterioration occurs, *terminate the tachycardia with a DC shock* before commencing drug therapy.

In emergencies, remember that some paroxysms can be terminated by a powerful thump over the lower sternum, so always try this first.

A few patients with good cardiac reserve have no symptoms and may require no treatment.

Ventricular Fibrillation

In this condition, purposeful ventricular contraction is replaced by irregular, uncoordinated and ineffective writhing of the ventricular myocardium. The ventricles neither fill nor empty and cardiac output suddenly ceases.

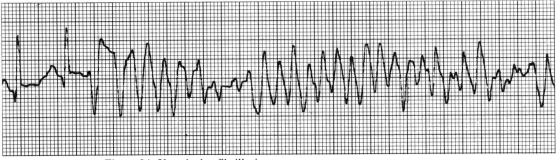

Figure 94. Ventricular fibrillation.

AETIOLOGY

Occurrence and causes
Commonly:
- following acute myocardial infarction or ischaemic attacks in patients with coronary heart disease
- as a terminal manifestation in any type of organic disease
- during surgical procedures under general anaesthesia
- as a result of electrocution, drowning or hypothermia
- as a toxic effect of drugs, e.g. digitalis, quinidine or isoprenaline

Rarely, in self-terminating paroxysms.

The occasional cause of Adams–Stokes attacks in complete heart block.

DIAGNOSIS

Ventricular fibrillation (VF) is the commonest cause of sudden death and should be assumed if the patient appears dead, is pulseless and has no heart sounds.

ECG

The ECG shows broad, bizarre, undulating complexes of varying amplitude and rate, but usually in the region of 300 per minute (Figure 94).

TREATMENT

Immediate treatment is essential, because permanent brain damage occurs after three or four minutes without effective cardiac output.

Do not wait for ECG proof of VF. If the patient is not already attached to an ECG machine, *start cardiopulmonary resuscitation without a moment's delay*. This is a situation where seconds count. A DC defibrillator usually restores normal rhythm without much difficulty.

If no defibrillator is immediately available, closed chest cardiac massage and artificial ventilation should be given until help arrives. Remember always, first to give the lower end of the sternum one or two firm blows with the clenched fist: this is sometimes effective in terminating the abnormal rhythm (Figure 95).

If treatment is successful, suppressive therapy should be considered to prevent recurrence (see Ventricular Tachycardia, page 79).

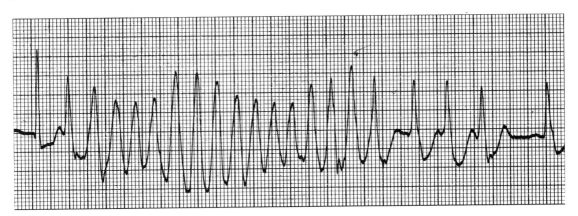

Figure 95. VF terminated by blow to lower sternum.

Ventricular Standstill (Asystole)

This is a condition in which the ventricles are motionless and there is no evidence of either electrical or mechanical ventricular activity. It is often referred to as asystolic cardiac arrest.

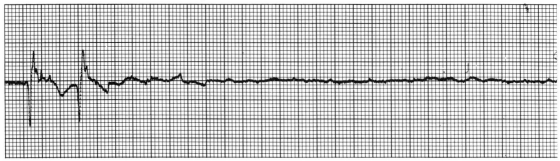

Figure 96. Ventricular standstill.

AETIOLOGY

Ventricular standstill is a frequent terminal event in many illnesses, especially in patients with heart disease. It is also a common cause of *late* death following myocardial infarction, when cardiac arrest is often asystolic. It may start with ventricular fibrillation and progress spontaneously to asystole, or be converted to asystole by a DC shock.

DIAGNOSIS

Asystole cannot be distinguished from ventricular fibrillation at the bedside without an ECG.

ECG

The ECG shows absence of QRS complexes on an undulating iso-electric line that may or may not be interrupted by P waves (Figure 96).

TREATMENT

Ventricular standstill is nearly always fatal. A viable rhythm may occasionally be restored by injecting 10ml of 1 in 10,000 adrenalin and 10ml 10% calcium chloride directly into the heart through the chest wall and then instituting cardiac pacing, during attempts at resuscitation.

Agonal Rhythm

Agonal rhythm is the ECG record of a dying heart that has ceased to function mechanically. The ECG shows grossly widened and distorted QRS complexes that occur irregularly and with gradually decreasing frequency until all electrical activity has ceased (Figure 97).

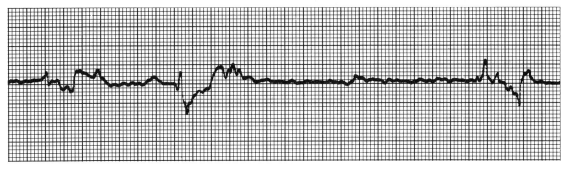

Figure 97. Agonal rhythm.

DISORDERS OF CONDUCTION

Sinus Block and Arrest

In this condition, the sinus impulse either fails to arise (sinus arrest) or fails to emerge from the sinus node (SA block). As a consequence, the atria are not activated and no impulse arrives at the junctional tissues to activate the ventricles.

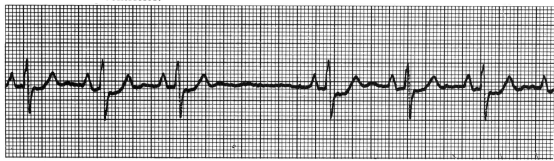

Figure 98. Sinus arrest.

AETIOLOGY

Physiological
- in sensitive individuals, vagal stimulation may suppress the SA node

Pathological
- myocardial infarction
- ischaemia
- rheumatic fever
- acute infections

Pharmacological
- digitalis
- quinidine
- salicylates

DIAGNOSIS

Sinus arrest is relatively uncommon, and of little clinical significance, except when an already slow heart rate is suddenly halved by the development of 2:1 SA block.

ECG

The ECG shows absent P, QRS and T waves between two normal complexes. The distance between them is at least twice the sinus cycle (Figure 98).

Sometimes, the pause is followed by an escape beat rather than the next sinus beat (Figure 99).

A very early P occurring on the T wave that precedes a pause, and whose conduction is blocked, may be mistaken for a sinus arrest (Figure 100).

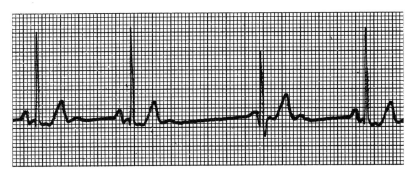

Figure 99. Sinus arrest followed by a junctional (nodal) escape beat.

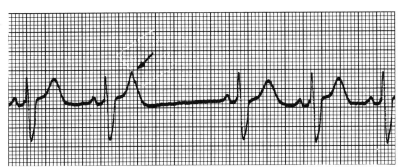

Figure 100. Early P (on T) with blocked conduction simulating sinus arrest.

TREATMENT

As a rule no treatment is required unless the block is pharmacologically induced.

If a slow heart rate is causing symptoms, the patient should be given atropine (see page 124). If this is ineffective, artificial pacing may occasionally be necessary.

In acute temporary arrest, cardiac resuscitation may be necessary, till normal rhythm returns spontaneously.

Sick Sinus Syndrome

This is a condition in which episodes of sinus node depression may alternate with paroxysms of rapid atrial rhythms. It is sometimes referred to as the tachycardia/bradycardia syndrome.

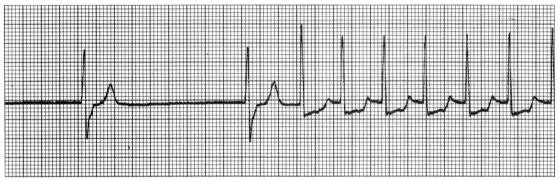

Figure 101. Sick sinus syndrome.

AETIOLOGY

Occurrence
It affects all age groups, but is commonest in the elderly.

Cause
No specific cause has been demonstrated; it is probably multifactorial.

DIAGNOSIS

The condition is often not recognised for what it is, because, unless the patient's visit coincides with an episode of bradycardia or tachycardia, examination of the cardiovascular system and a routine ECG reveal no abnormality. The symptoms should arouse suspicion, and the availability of 24-hour tape-recording has greatly assisted with diagnosis.

Symptoms

Some have no symptoms, some have palpitation, some have symptoms suggesting a low cardiac output such as fatigue, breathlessness and light-headedness, and some present with syncopal attacks or convulsions.

Pulse and heart rate

The pulse and heart rate may be normal during examination. Sometimes it is abnormally slow or abnormally rapid.

ECG

The routine ECG is often normal. It, or a tape, may show any type of sinus node depression (bradycardia, prolonged pauses, arrest or block) or any type of atrial tachycardia, flutter or fibrillation interspersed with long or short periods of what appears to be normal sinus rhythm (Figure 101).

TREATMENT

Only patients with troublesome or dangerous symptoms should be treated. The condition should not be treated because it is there.

Warning
Patients who do not require treatment when first seen should be kept under surveillance, because this condition is generally progressive. Troublesome tachycardia requires antidysrhythmic therapy (see pages 54–55). Low output states require cardiac pacing (see page 142). Sometimes both are required in the same patient, because increasing the slow rate by pacing does not necessarily prevent runs of tachycardia (Figure 102).

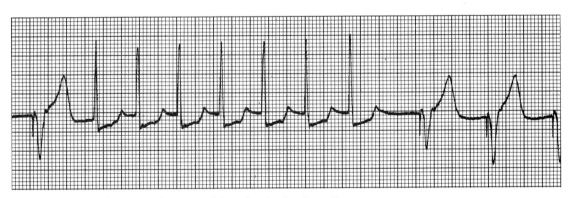

Figure 102. Tachycardia despite successful pacing for bradycardia.

Atrioventricular Block

Atrioventricular block is classified into three degrees:
- in *first degree block* conduction through the junctional tissues is delayed, but all the supraventricular impulses reach the ventricles, albeit somewhat slowly
- in *second degree block* some supraventricular impulses may be delayed in reaching the ventricles, and some may never reach the ventricles
- in *third degree block* no supraventricular impulses reach the ventricles

First and second degree block are often referred to as partial heart block. Third degree block is usually referred to as complete heart block. The term *high grade* is still frequently used when referring to second and third degree block.

Some patients progress from normal sinus rhythm through all degrees of block to complete block, but in practice any degree of block may be encountered without prior or subsequent evidence of the others.

First Degree AV block

First degree heart block is present when the AV conduction time is prolonged to more than 0.20 seconds (Figure 103).

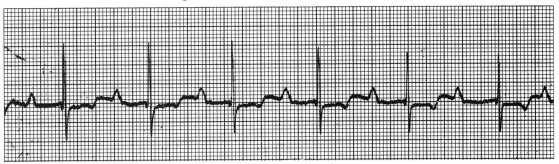

Figure 103. First degree heart block.

AETIOLOGY

The site of the block is usually within the AV node.

Occurrence and causes
Occasionally in apparently healthy people.

More frequently:
* in infectious diseases
  – rheumatic fever
  – diphtheria
  – myocarditis
* in elderly patients with
  – ischaemia or
  – fibrosis of the conducting tissues

Commonly:
* as a transient phenomenon after myocardial infarction
* in overdosage with digitalis

DIAGNOSIS

In infections it may act as an indicator of severity. In ischaemia or fibrosis it acts as a warning that more serious block may occur.

89

Symptoms

First degree block causes no symptoms.

Pause and heart rate

The pulse and heart rate are not affected.

ECG

The PR interval is seen to be more than 0.20 seconds in duration.

TREATMENT

No specific treatment is required unless it is caused by too much digitalis. In these circumstances the drug should be discontinued until normal conduction is restored.

Second Degree AV Block

Second degree heart block is classified as Type I or Type II and is much more complex and difficult to understand than either first degree block or third degree block.

Second Degree Block-Type I

In this type of second degree heart block (often referred to as Wenckebach block), delay through the junctional tissues increases progressively with each beat until an impulse is completely blocked. Following a pause due to the resulting absent ventricular contraction, the cycle repeats itself.

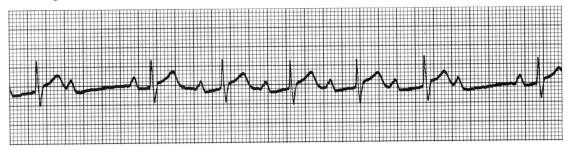

Figure 104. Wenckebach block.

AETIOLOGY

Occurrence
Frequently in acute illnesses such as myocardial infarction and infections. Usually transient.

Causes
Particularly:
- inferior infarction
- rheumatic fever
- diptheria
- toxic effects of digitalis

DIAGNOSIS

Symptoms
None.

Pulse and heart rate
The condition should be suspected clinically when three, four, five or more beats are followed by a pause and this sequence repeats itself, possibly with slight variations.

ECG
The diagnosis can only be made with certainty when the ECG shows progressive lengthening of the PR interval in successive complexes until a P wave is not followed by a QRS (Figure 104).

TREATMENT

This type of second degree block is relatively benign. It seldom progresses to complete heart block and even if it does, a relatively rapid junctional escape rhythm usually takes over because the site of block is high in the junctional tissues. It should, however, warn of the possibility that more serious abnormalities may arise.

No specific treatment is required unless it is caused by too much digitalis.

Second Degree Block-Type II

In this type of second degree heart block, beats are dropped without preceding lengthening of the conduction time through the junctional tissues. The dropped beats may occur:
- randomly and without warning
- in regular sequence (2:1 block where every second impulse fails to reach the ventricle; less often 3:1, 4:1 etc.)

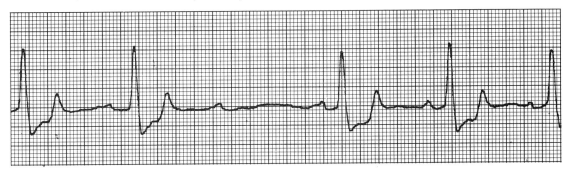

Figure 105. Randomly without warning.

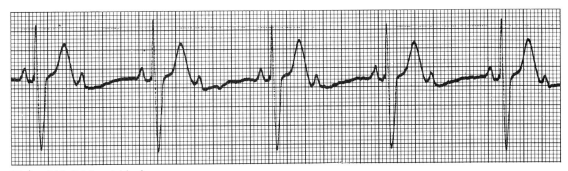

Figure 106. 2:1 heart block.

AETIOLOGY

Occurrence
Much less common than Type I second degree block.

Random dropped beats are seen mainly in patients with recent myocardial infarction. This is a serious abnormality of conduction because the block occurs in the bundle of His or distal to it, with the result that if it becomes complete, a subsidiary pacemaker may either fail to emerge or have a very slow rate.

93

2 (or more):1 block is seen mainly following recent myocardial infarction or in chronic degenerative disease of the conducting system. It is less serious than randomly dropped beats because the block usually occurs in the AV node, with the result that if it becomes complete, a reasonably rapid pacemaker takes over.

DIAGNOSIS

Symptoms

Single dropped beats cause no symptoms and are unlikely to be noticed by the patient.

2 (or more):1 block slows the heart rate, and symptoms of low output may occur if it becomes very slow.

Pulse and heart rate

Single dropped beats are easily detected. With slow rates an exact diagnosis can only be made with the help of an ECG.

ECG

With dropped beats, occasional P waves are not followed by QRS complexes (Figure 105). The PR interval of the conducted beats is constant and may be either normal or prolonged, i.e. patients with first degree block may also drop beats. When the PR interval is prolonged, it often shortens in the first beat following the pause.

With 2:1 block, two P waves are seen between each QRS complex (Figure 106). With 3:1 block, three P waves are seen between each QRS complex. With 4:1 block, four P waves are seen between each QRS complex. In each case the PR interval of the conducted beat is constant.

Occasionally, several types of block may co-exist, e.g. 2:1 block with a long PR interval and occasional dropped beats.

TREATMENT

Note. Patients developing second degree block following myocardial infarction must be observed very carefully.

In inferior infarction, they should be treated only if the heart rate becomes too slow to maintain an adequate cardiac output or the QRS complexes become broadened. In these circumstances atropine should be given and repeated if necessary. If the response is inadequate or the patient's condition deteriorates, a temporary pacemaker should be inserted.

In anterior infarction, second degree block is a sign of extensive myocardial damage and a temporary pacing catheter should be inserted without delay. If extreme bradycardia occurs, isoprenaline should be given until the pacemaker is functioning satisfactorily.

Bundle Branch Blocks

Any interruption to the passage of impulses down either the right or left branches of the bundle of His causes delayed conduction through some parts of the ventricles and an abnormal sequence of activation. Complete interruption produces broadening of the QRS complexes to more than 0.12 seconds and characteristic ECG patterns known as right and left bundle branch block (see Figure 3, 'The conduction system').

Right Bundle Branch Block

When the right bundle branch is blocked, activation is delayed because impulses have to spread across to the right ventricle from the left ventricle. This results in abnormal QRS complexes characterised by a broad rsR pattern in the right precordial leads (Figure 107).

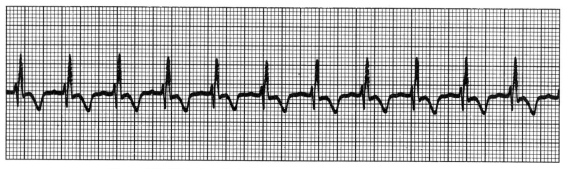

Figure 107. Right bundle branch block.

AETIOLOGY

In adults, right bundle branch block is usually due to coronary heart disease. Sometimes, it is seen as a transient pattern following acute pulmonary embolism. In children, it may be an isolated congenital lesion, but is more commonly associated with other congenital cardiac malformations, notably atrial septal defects.

DIAGNOSIS

Right bundle branch block is an ECG diagnosis, but it may be suspected if the pulmonary and aortic components of the second heart sound are widely split.

It is usually of no clinical significance except to warn of possible heart disease or, following recent myocardial infarction, the onset of complete heart block, if it is accompanied by left axis deviation.

TREATMENT

No treatment is required.

96

Left Bundle Branch Block

When the left bundle is blocked, the septum is activated from right to left instead of from left to right. Activation is delayed, because impulses have to spread across to the left ventricle from the right ventricle. This results in abnormal QRS complexes, characterised by loss of the initial Q waves and by broad, mainly positive deflections in the left precordial leads (Figure 108).

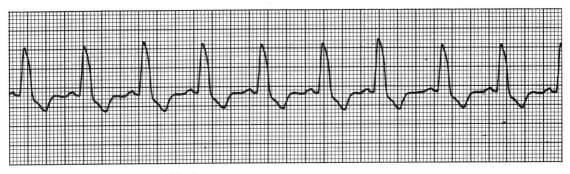

Figure 108. Left bundle branch block.

AETIOLOGY

Left bundle branch block is rarely seen in normal hearts. It is usually a sign of coronary heart disease, but may occur in any disease involving the left ventricle.

DIAGNOSIS

Like right bundle branch block it is an ECG diagnosis, but is seldom suspected clinically.

TREATMENT

No treatment is required.

Hemiblock (Fascicular Block)

Soon after it leaves the bundle of His, the *left bundle branch* divides into several fascicles. The two main divisions of fascicles (anterior and posterior) supply the anterosuperior and the postero-inferior parts of the left ventricle. If either is blocked, the sequence of activation in the electrically dominant left ventricle is altered. This produces a characteristic ECG pattern known as **hemiblock** or **fascicular block**.

In left anterior hemiblock, the postero-inferior part of the ventricle is activated first and the ECG shows left axis deviation. In left posterior hemiblock, the anterosuperior part of the ventricle is activated first and the ECG shows right axis deviation.

In both, there are also subtle and somewhat complex changes in the nature of the QRS complexes in the limb and precordial leads.

Fascicular block

The concept that within the bundle of His, the left branch has two main fascicles has caused the *right bundle branch* to be regarded as the third fascicle; hence the **bifascicular** and **trifascicular block**.

Bifascicular block is said to be present when the right bundle (fascicle) and either of the main left fascicles are failing to conduct.

Trifascicular block is a term sometimes used to describe complete heart block when all three fascicles have become blocked individually rather than collectively, as happens more commonly when the lesion is higher in the AV junctional tissues.

These blocks usually occur acutely following recent myocardial infarction. They are ECG diagnoses and are used mainly as criteria for pacing the heart in coronary care units.

Third Degree AV Block (Complete Block)

In this condition the block in the AV junctional tissues is complete. No conduction between the atria and ventricles is possible, and they function independently of one another under the control of separate pacemakers.

The atria usually remain in normal sinus rhythm, although any of the atrial dysrhythmias may be present or there may be little or no sign of atrial activity. The ventricles usually maintain a slow idioventricular rhythm with broad QRS complexes but, if the site of the block is above the bifurcation of the His bundle, the QRS complexes have a more normal appearance.

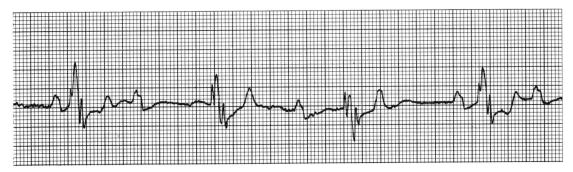

Figure 109. Complete heart block.

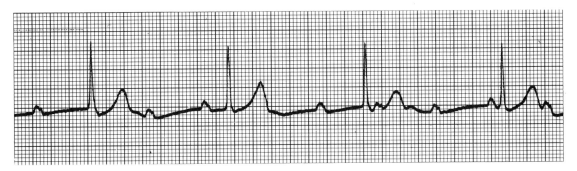

Figure 110. Complete heart block.

AETIOLOGY

Complete heart block occurs in acute and chronic forms. When acute, it is usually temporary; when chronic, it is usually permanent.

Acute complete heart block
Usually a complication of myocardial infarction.
Occasionally a temporary complication of myocarditis or diptheria.

Chronic complete heart block
Usually a sclerodegenerative disease in the elderly.

Occasionally seen in coronary heart disease or infiltrative diseases such as:
• calcific aortic stenosis
• sarcoidosis
• Hodgkin's disease
• trauma, including surgery

Rarely, it is congenital.

DIAGNOSIS

Symptoms

These depend to a large extent upon the ventricular rate and the state of the myocardium.

Some patients have no symptoms, some are merely aware of a slow powerful heart beat and some (usually those with a very slow heart rate) complain of fatigue, lightheadedness and symptoms of heart failure.

Those who are having Adams–Stokes seizures with drop attacks due to sudden, temporary loss of consciousness show evidence of physical injury.

Pulse and heart rate

The pulse and heart rates are slow, regular and equal, varying from 25–50 per minute and showing little or no response to exercise. The arterial pulse is of large volume. Cannon waves are often seen in the jugular venous pulse. The intensity of the first heart sound varies and atrial sounds are sometimes heard over the precordium.

ECG

The ECG shows slow, regular, broad, bizarre QRS complexes that often resemble ventricular ectopic beats (Figure 109). Sometimes, when the pacemaker is high in the junctional tissues, they have a more normal appearance (Figure 110).

The P waves occur regularly at a much faster rate than the QRS complexes and are unrelated to them. If the block occurs as a complication of acute myocardial infarction in a patient with sinus tachycardia, the atrial rate remains fairly rapid (Figure 110). If the sinus rate varies (for example, with respiration), the PP interval varies; and sometimes the interval between successive P waves is shortened when a QRS complex intervenes between them (Figure 57). In some cases, no P waves are visible.

Adams–Stokes seizures are nearly always caused by ventricular asystole. During an attack, no QRS complexes are seen on the record. The P waves, if present, continue as before (Figure 111). Occasionally, the seizure is precipitated by a burst of very rapid ventricular tachycardia or a short period of ventricular fibrillation.

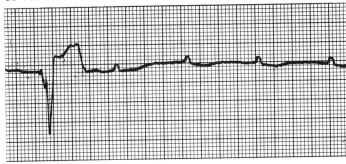

Figure 111.
Onset of an Adams-Stokes attack.

TREATMENT

This depends upon the cause of the block and whether or not it is likely to be permanent. With a few exceptions, treatment should be on account of symptoms and not because the patient has heart block.

Acute block following myocardial infarction

With inferior infarction, the patient should only be treated if the heart block is causing haemodynamic problems or if the QRS complexes become broadened.

With anterior infarction, a temporary pacemaker should be inserted immediately.

Chronic block

If the patient has a low cardiac output or is having Adams–Stokes seizures, a permanent pacemaker should be inserted to:
- relieve symptoms by increasing the heart rate (Figure 112)
- increase life expectancy
- decrease dependency on others.

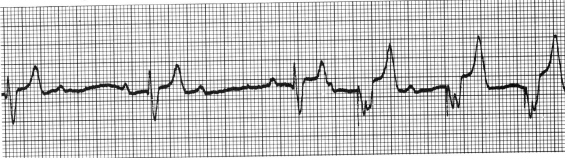

Figure 112. Slow idioventricular heart rate of 39 per minute increased to 68 by pacing.

Following pacing, the activity of the intrinsic cardiac pacemakers varies within wide limits. This has important therapeutic implications if for any reason the artificial pacemaker fails to function. In some cases the complete block continues as it did before pacing was commenced. In some cases there is very slow idioventricular rhythm with no P waves. In some cases there are regular P waves but no QRS complexes. In some cases there is no sign of spontaneous activity in either the atria or the ventricles (Figures 113–116).

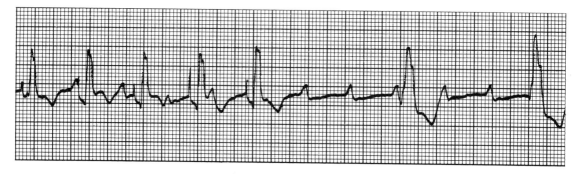

Figure 113. Complete heart block.

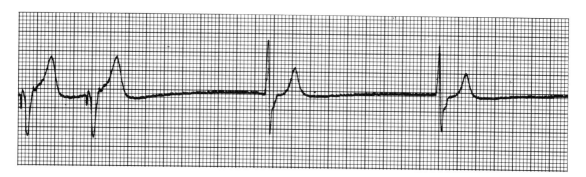

Figure 114. Very slow ventricular rhythm with no P waves.

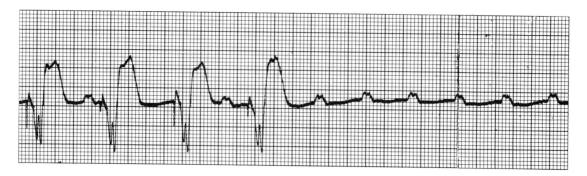

Figure 115. Regular P waves but no QRS complexes.

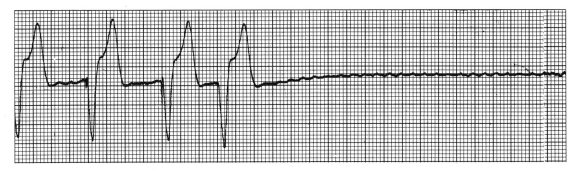

Figure 116. Neither P waves nor QRS complexes.

Adams–Stokes seizures

These may occur without provocation and without warning at any time, either at rest or on exertion. They are most commonly seen in the elderly. The attacks are nearly always self-terminating and although seldom lasting more than 10–30 seconds, often cause injury when the unconscious patient falls to the ground. If spontaneous recovery does not occur, the usual procedures for treating cardiac arrest should be followed (see page 128).

Atrioventricular Dissociation

This is a condition in which the atria and the ventricles function independently of each other, not because there is anything intrinsically wrong with the AV conducting tissues that prevents impulses passing through them, but because the atria and the ventricles are under the control of separate pacemakers. Neither pacemaker captures the other's territory because each is initiating impulses almost simultaneously and the territory of one is always refractory to stimulation by the other.

AV dissociation, unlike heart block, is always secondary to some other abnormality of pacemaker function. If circumstances change and the pacemakers become sufficiently out of phase, one of them usually captures both territories.

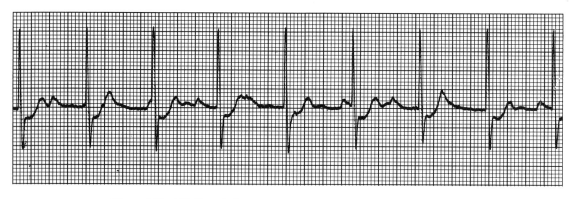

Figure 117. AV dissociation.

AETIOLOGY

Occurrence and causes
Most commonly a temporary disturbance following myocardial infarction or a toxic effect of digitalis

Occasionally:
- caused by excessive vagal stimulation
- a complication of acute infections, such as pneumonia, diphtheria or typhoid

DIAGNOSIS

AV dissociation is seldom diagnosed clinically, because the heart rate is usually within the normal range. It may be suspected when the intensity of the first heart sound varies and occasional cannon waves are seen in the jugular venous pulse.

ECG

An ECG is essential for diagnosis. The P waves and the QRS complexes occur at almost the same rate, but bear no relationship to each other (Figure 117).

The ventricular pacemaker, which is usually in the AV tissues, is, as a rule, a little faster than the supraventricular pacemaker. As a result, successive P waves are often seen to overtake (walk through) the QRS complexes; they start off in front of them, then become lost within them and finally reappear behind them (Figure 118).

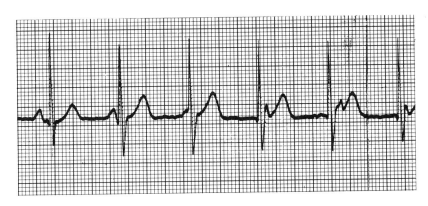

Figure 118. P waves 'walking through' the QRS complexes.

TREATMENT

No specific treatment is required, other than for the primary condition.

Pre-Excitation (WPW Syndrome)

Pre-excitation occurs when a sinus impulse bypasses the normal conducting pathway through the AV junctional tissues and activates the ventricles sooner than would have been possible had it travelled through them in the usual way.

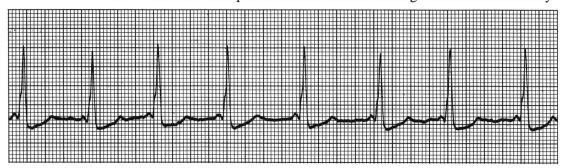

Figure 119. Pre-excitation.

AETIOLOGY

Occurrence
Usually in healthy young adults without evidence of heart disease but liable to attacks of paroxysmal tachycardia (the Wolff–Parkinson–White syndrome).

Occasionally in patients with organic heart disease.

Causes
The bypass may be:
- across a myocardial bridge between the atria and ventricles
- through abnormal fibres in the AV junctional tissues

Incidence
Difficult to determine, but likely to be only one in several thousand. It has received much more attention than it merits, because of its interest to electrophysiologists.

DIAGNOSIS

Symptoms

Pre-excitation itself causes no symptoms. Most cases present with paroxysmal tachycardia or are discovered when an ECG is recorded for some other reason.

Pulse and heart rate

The pulse and heart rate are normal unless the patient is seen during a paroxysm of tachycardia.

Such paroxysms are usually of supraventricular tachycardia. Sometimes they are of atrial fibrillation or atrial flutter and occasionally a severe ventricular dysrythmia that may be fatal.

ECG

The ECG shows a short PR interval of 0.10 seconds or less. The QRS complexes are correspondingly broadened, usually by a slurred upstroke of the R wave due to a delta wave caused by early ventricular activation via the bypass (Figure 119).

The delta waves often disappear during paroxysms of tachycardia, and the QRS complexes are of normal width (Figure 120).

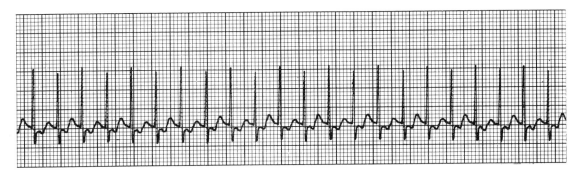

Figure 120. Loss of pre-excitation during a paroxysm of rapid supraventricular tachycardia.

TREATMENT

The paroxysms of tachycardia are usually of the re-entrant type and often respond to treatment in the normal way. Sometimes it is easier to prevent them than to treat them, and in such cases carefully designed prophylactic therapy is important.

Beta blockers, digoxin or verapamil can be used to slow conduction through the AV node.

If the ventricular rate is very rapid, IV verapamil or a DC shock may be required to restore normal rhythm.

Note. Digoxin has recently been reported occasionally to cause ventricular fibrillation.

Never give IV verapamil to patients who have recently had digoxin or beta blockers: it may cause asystolic arrest.

4

SPOT THE DIAGNOSIS

Here are some examples of disorders that you should now be able to recognise. The diagnosis in each case is on page 116.

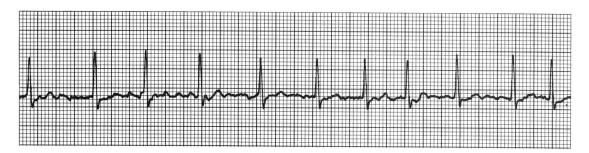

Figure 121.

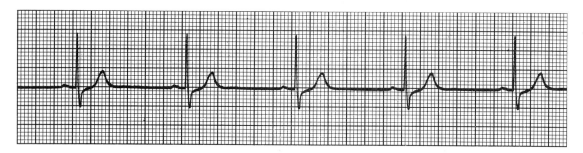

Figure 122.

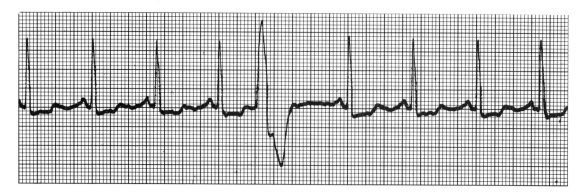

Figure 123.

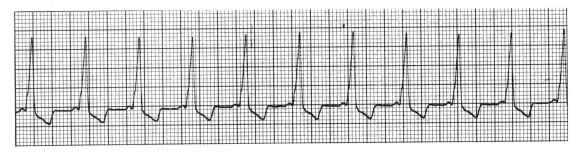

Figure 124.

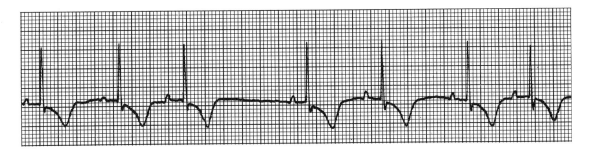

Figure 125.

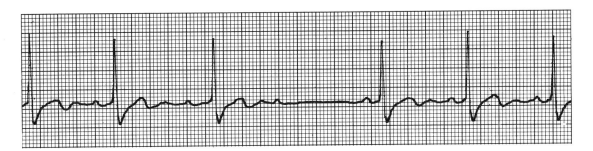

Figure 126.

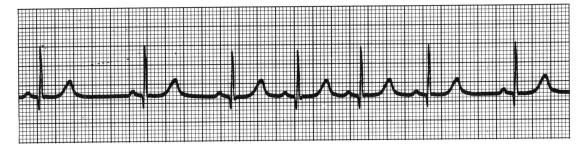

Figure 127.

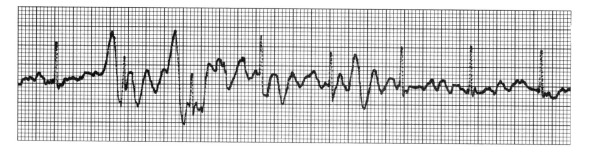

Figure 128.

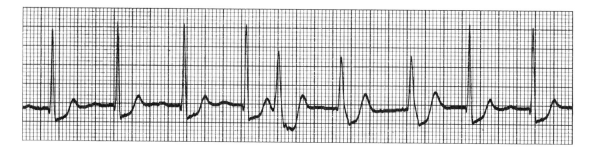

Figure 129.

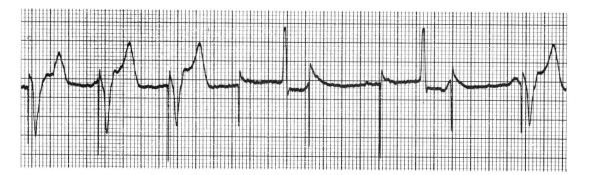

Figure 130.

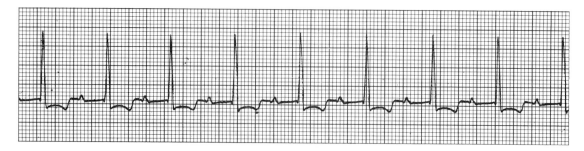

Figure 131.

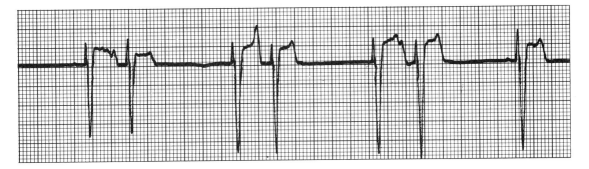

Figure 132.

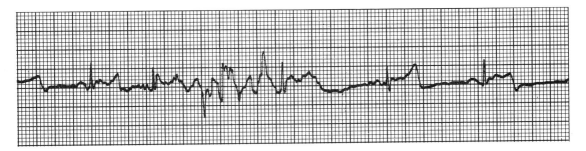

Figure 133.

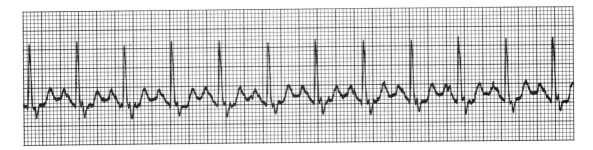

Figure 134.

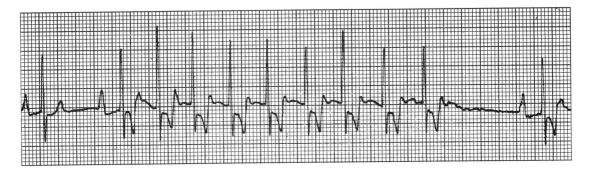

Figure 135.

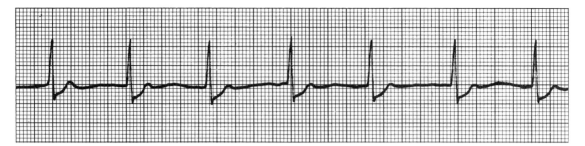

Figure 136.

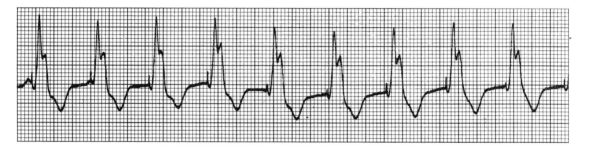

Figure 137.

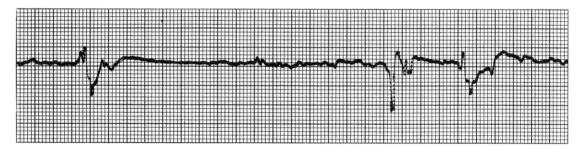

Figure 138.

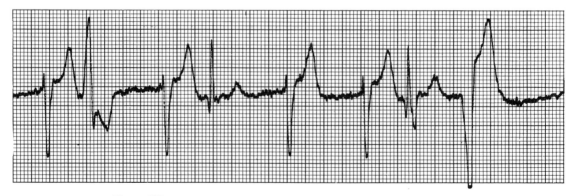

Figure 139.

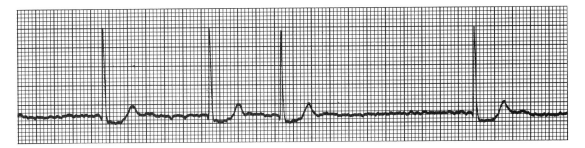

Figure 140.

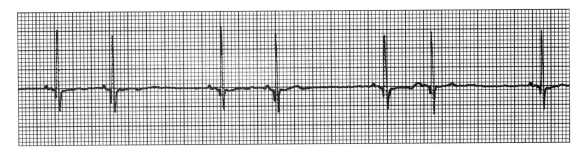

Figure 141.

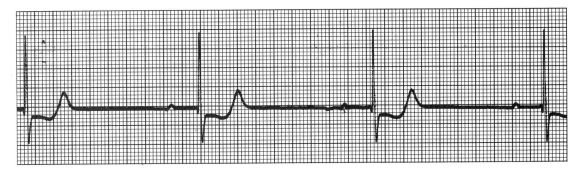

Figure 142.

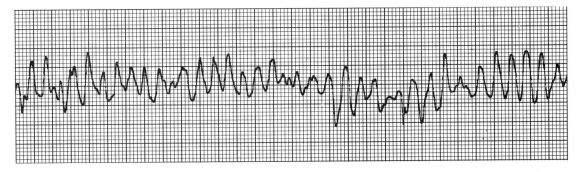

Figure 143.

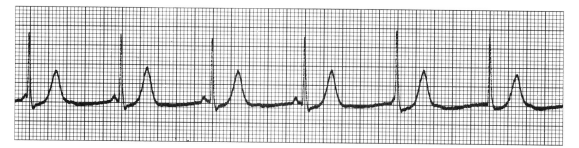

Figure 144.

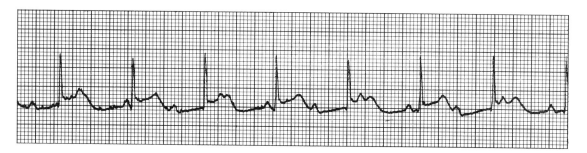

Figure 145.

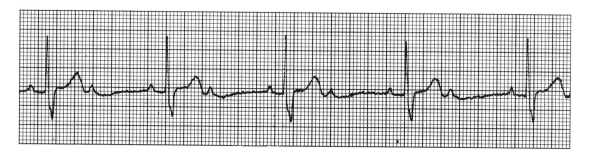

Figure 146.

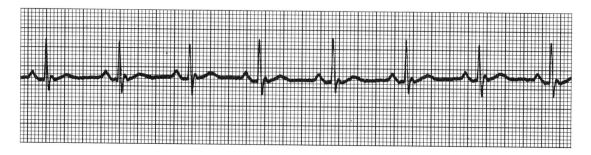

Figure 147.

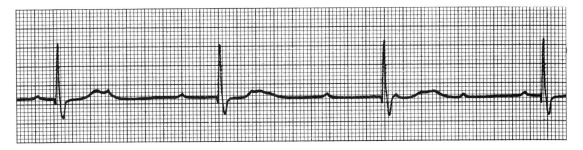

Figure 148.

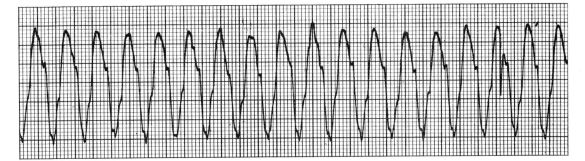

Figure 149.

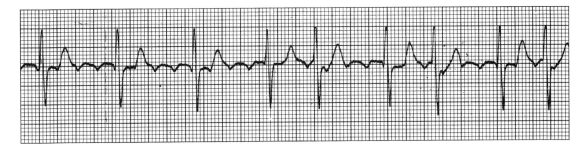

Figure 150.

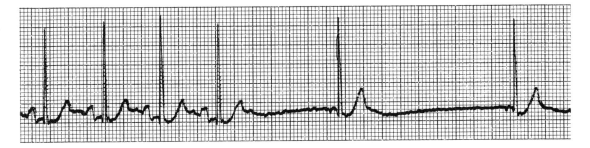

Figure 151.

Figure 121. Atrial fibrillation.

Figure 122. Sinus bradycardia.

Figure 123. Ventricular ectopic beat.

Figure 124. Pre-excitation.

Figure 125. Sinus arrest.

Figure 126. 2nd degree heart block (Wenckebach).

Figure 127. Sinus dysrhythmia.

Figure 128. Loose lead artefact.

Figure 129. A pacemaker failing to capture the heart.

Figure 130. R on T ventricular ectopic beat, initiating a short run of idioventricular rhythm.

Figure 131. 1st degree heart block.

Figure 132. Reciprocal beats.

Figure 133. Patient movement artefact.

Figure 134. Sinus tachycardia.

Figure 135. A short paroxysm of supraventricular tachycardia.

Figure 136. Junctional rhythm.

Figure 137. A heart being paced.

Figure 138. Agonal rhythm.

Figure 139. Multifocal ventricular ectopic beats.

Figure 140. Atrial fibrillation.

Figure 141. Supraventricular ectopic beats, causing coupled rhythm.

Figure 142. Extreme bradycardia with 1st degree heart block.

Figure 143. Ventricular fibrillation.

Figure 144. Wandering pacemaker.

Figure 145. AV dissociation.

Figure 146. 2:1 heart block.

Figure 147. Sinus rhythm.

Figure 148. Complete heart block.

Figure 149. Ventricular tachycardia.

Figure 150. Atrial flutter.

Figure 151. Tachycardia/bradycardia syndrome.

5

TREATMENT

The advent of coronary care units has given great impetus to the search for new, more effective and safer antidysrhythmic therapy.

Several promising drugs have been introduced during the last few years. Although they have made treatment more effective:

- none has proved to be ideal
- all are potentially harmful
- most can cause unpleasant side effects
- some may even be lethal when given in excessive amounts or together with other powerful agents.

PHARMACOLOGICAL ACTION

Drugs in current use act in a variety of ways. Many of them have more than one action.

Despite their potentially beneficial effects, most of them also depress myocardial function. They should, therefore, be used with caution and only when absolutely necessary, particularly in patients who have had other antidysrhythmic drugs.

It is currently fashionable to classify them according to their predominant electrophysiological properties.

Class I drugs (disopyramide, lignocaine, mexiletine, phenytoin, procainamide, quinidine, tocainide):

- impede sodium transport across cell membranes
- slow the rapid phase of depolarisation (phase 0)
- reduce the extent of overshoot

Some possess local anaesthetic properties that stabilise membranes.

Class II drugs (beta blockers):

- are taken up at sympathetic nerve endings
- antagonise beta-adrenergic receptors
- interfere with noradrenaline release

Class III drugs (amiodarone, sotalol):

- prolong the repolarisation phase of the action potential
- increase the refractory period of myocardial fibres

117

Class IV drugs (verapamil):

- interfere with calcium movement and depress phases 2 and 3 of the action potential

Such classifications, which are based on laboratory experiments, are helpful in understanding how the various drugs work. In practice, it is probably more helpful to classify them according to their site of action:

(a) drugs that act on the atria and slow conduction through the junctional tissues (e.g. beta blockers, digoxin, verapamil),
(b) drugs that act on the ventricles (e.g. lignocaine, mexiletine, phenytoin, tocainide, some beta blockers),
(c) drugs that act on both the atria and the ventricles (e.g. amiodarone, disopyramide, procainamide, quinidine).

Because of their different modes and sites of action, some drugs are more suitable than others in the treatment of specific disorders. For example:
- those reducing excitability are used to dampen ectopic activity
- those depressing conduction are used to slow ventricular response to supraventricular stimuli

Examples

Rapid atrial rhythms may be:
- prevented by suppressing the ectopic beats that initiate them
- terminated by re-establishing sinus rhythm
- made less troublesome by slowing conduction through the AV junctional tissues

Rapid junctional rhythms are mostly of the re-entrant type and can be:
- controlled by prolonging AV recovery time
- prevented by suppressing ectopic activity

Rapid ventricular rhythms usually occur following myocardial infarction. When life-threatening they can be:
- terminated immediately, using a DC shock

Otherwise they can be:
- treated with any drug that has a specific effect on ventricular potentials. This includes most of those in current use and is often a process of trial and error
- prevented either by suppressing the ectopic activity that triggers them or making the ventricular myocardium less excitable

SIDE EFFECTS

The problem of side effects remains unsolved. With many drugs such as digoxin, disopyramide, mexiletine and quinidine, side effects are closely related to the amount prescribed and can be minimised or abolished by careful control of the dose and the frequency of administration.

With others such as practolol and procainamide, the drug appears to act as a trigger substance and can sometimes cause or initiate irreversible damage, unless given over a very short period.

THERAPEUTIC PRINCIPLES

Having taken a careful history, examined the patient and recorded an ECG, the first thing to do is to decide about:
- the likely nature of the abnormality
- the presence or absence of underlying heart disease

Having done this, you must then decide whether or not treatment is really necessary.

In many cases, the disorder is of little or no consequence and no treatment is required, apart from reassurance and a simple explanation of what is happening.

If the disorder is more troublesome, a decision whether or not to treat may depend upon:
- the frequency of attacks
- their severity
- the patient's reaction to them

Treatment can be used to:
- prevent or suppress ectopic beats that may initiate ectopic rhythms
- prevent or suppress paroxysms of tachycardia
- slow the ventricular response to rapid supraventricular stimuli if they cannot be prevented or suppressed
- increase the heart rate when it is too slow

When the abnormal rhythm cannot easily be abolished, it is often wise to accept it and concentrate therapy on maintaining a normal ventricular rate.

Keep in mind that:

- symptoms are often evanescent and may subside spontaneously without treatment
- whenever possible, it is better to treat the cause of the symptoms than the symptoms themselves
- the side effects of the drugs used may be more unpleasant than the symptoms for which they are being prescribed
- patients on treatment should keep a diary of their symptoms so that the effects of the treatment may be assessed objectively

- treatment should be stopped periodically to make sure that it is still necessary
- if emergency treatment is required to save life, *immediate action based on probability takes priority over all else.* Do not allow a patient to die from ventricular fibrillation while waiting for an ECG to prove it!

When a patient is referred to hospital or discharged from hospital, remember to indicate the name of the drug and the dose prescribed to those who will be providing continuous care.

DRUG THERAPY

Most disorders can now be controlled with carefully chosen and well directed drug therapy. Of the drugs used:
- many are powerful substances with complex and sometimes paradoxical modes of action
- some will cure disorders in one concentration, and cause them in another
- most can produce unwanted side effects that may be unpleasant, unacceptable or dangerous

As their effects and side effects vary from patient to patient, therapy is most likely to be successful if it is firmly based upon a sound knowledge of their mode of action and the patient's likely reaction to them.

Which drug should be used?

If treatment is really necessary, most disorders are usually either very easy to control or very difficult to control.

With the growing choice of drugs available, the treatment of difficult cases should be by well-informed trial and error. So, warn the patient that the first drug tried may not turn out to be the most suitable or the most effective of those that are available.

If the disorder responds, but the drug causes unacceptable side effects, use another drug with the same mode of action that has potentially different side effects.

If the disorder does not respond, use another drug with a different mode of action.

Sometimes a combination of actions is required to achieve the desired effect, and this may not be possible with one drug.

Example

In a rapid supraventricular tachycardia, the junctional tissues may not be able to conduct all the impulses arriving at the AV node. As a result, the ventricular rate is slower than the atrial rate.

When a drug is used to slow the atrial rate, the junctional tissues may then be able to conduct all the impulses. As a result, the ventricular rate (heart rate) is faster after treatment than it was before it.

It is then necessary also to slow the rate of conduction through the junctional tissues by:

- adding a drug possessing this property, or
- changing to a drug that possesses both the required properties, i.e. one that slows the atrial rate and the rate of conduction through the junctional tissues.

Side effects

Unless there are special dangers, it is, as a rule, better to tell patients to report any symptoms that occur than to tell them what specific symptoms to look out for.

In the following pages therapeutic agents are listed alphabetically; their uses and possible side effects are discussed. Where appropriate, the pharmacopoeial or non-proprietary name is followed by the corresponding proprietary name in parentheses. Proprietary names are identified throughout by an initial capital letter.

Amiodarone
(Cordarone X)

ACTION

Amiodarone prolongs the duration of the action potential and the refractory period of the:
- atrial myocardium
- AV junctional tissues
- ventricular myocardium
- anomalous bypass tracts

Speed of action

It acts slowly (up to 4 weeks may be required to reach a full response), so no immediate benefit can be expected.

Its half-life is 14–28 days and some activity may persist for several months after treatment is discontinued.

INDICATIONS

Amiodarone is highly effective in:
- a wide variety of supraventricular and ventricular dysrhythmias
- reciprocating AV tachycardias associated with the WPW syndrome

but, because of frequent side effects that are sometimes serious and occasionally fatal, it should only be used for significant disorders in those who are unresponsive to other drugs; and then only after careful and expert evaluation.

CONTRAINDICATIONS

Give with caution to patients:
- whose heart rate is already slow
- who are fully digitalised, especially the elderly

ADMINISTRATION

Orally
Initially 600mg (3 × 200mg) a day for the first week; moving on to 400mg a day for the second week; then maintain on at least 200mg a day depending upon response (some patients require much less).

Intravenously
5mg/kg by slow infusion (20–120 minutes) in 250ml 5% dextrose. It should only be used under cardiological control in an intensive care unit.

SIDE EFFECTS

- bradycardia
- metallic taste in mouth, gastro-intestinal upset
- hepatitis
- photosensitivity and discoloration of skin
- peripheral neuropathy
- headaches, vertigo, sleeplessness, nightmares
- muscle weakness, fatigue
- pulmonary alveolitis
- corneal microdeposits

Amiodarone contains iodine; most patients show an increase in T_4 and free thyroxine index without developing clinical thyroid disease.

SUPERVISION AND FOLLOW UP

Because of its frequent side effects, some of which warrant withdrawal of treatment, patients taking amiodarone require careful supervision and regular follow up. Those on long-term treatment should have serial eye examinations.

Atropine Sulphate

ACTION

Atropine is a parasympathetic blocking agent. It blocks acetylcholine at the synaptic junctions and cholinergic nerve endings. Its main action is to:
- shorten the refractory period in AV junctional tissues
- counteract the effect of the vagus on AV conduction and impulse formation

INDICATIONS

Mainly used to accelerate the heart during transient episodes of severe sinus bradycardia often seen soon after myocardial infarction. If they last longer, it can be used to hold the line until other means of maintaining cardiac output are instituted. It has little relevance to practice outside coronary care units. It is occasionally used in SA block and partial heart block caused by para-sympathetic overactivity.

ADMINISTRATION

Atropine acts rapidly and is used for short-term therapy only. Initially, give 0.6mg intravenously. Repeat after 10 minutes and, if necessary, again after 30 minutes. Do not give more than 3mg in 24 hours.

Alternatively, it can be given subcutaneously or intramuscularly.

SIDE EFFECTS

Serious side effects are uncommon with normal doses. It often causes:
- a dry mouth
- difficulty with speech

Toxic doses cause:
- dilatation of pupils and visual impairment
- urinary retention
- confusion
- hallucinations

Beta Blockers

acebutolol (Sectral); atenolol (Tenormin); metoprolol (Betaloc, Lopresor); nadolol (Corgard); oxprenolol (Trasicor); pindolol (Visken); propranolol (Berkolol, Inderal); sotalol (Beta-Cardone, Sotacor); timolol (Betim, Blocadren)

All the currently available drugs in this group antagonise cardiac beta adrenoceptors, whether or not they are cardioselective. Any of them can be used to treat or prevent disorders of rate or rhythm. The ultimate choice often depends upon their side effects, which vary with their relative lipid solubility and partial agonist activity, rather than upon minor differences in their electrophysiological effects. Cardioselectivity is of little significance when considering a drug's clinical efficiency, but may have slightly more importance when considering its possible toxicity.

Most lipid-soluble	*Least lipid-soluble*	*Cardioselective (B_1)*
metoprolol	atenolol	acebutolol
oxprenolol	nadolol	atenolol
propranolol	sotalol	metoprolol
timolol		

Partial agonist activity (in descending order of potency)
pindolol
oxprenolol
acebutolol (also an alpha blocker)

ACTION

The beta adrenergic blocking agents affect rate, rhythm and conduction by:
- reversing the effects of sympathetic nerve stimulation and circulating catecholamines. This prevents shortening of the refractory period and an increase in automaticity and conduction velocity.
- direct action on myocardial cells. This increases the effective refractory period of the atrial myocardium and the AV junctional tissues. The effect on the His-Purkinje system and the ventricular myocardium is less marked.
- additionally sotalol has Class III activity that prolongs the duration of the action potential and increases the length of the refractory period.

INDICATIONS

Beta blockers are useful in the treatment of:

• supraventricular dysrhythmias	to suppress and prevent supra-ventricular and junctional ectopic rhythms
• a rapid ventricular response to supraventricular stimuli	to slow the ventricular rate in atrial fibrillation and flutter when digitalis alone fails to do so
• organic heart disease e.g. angina	to reduce rate response to emotion and exercise
• sinus tachycardia e.g. severe anxiety states, thyrotoxicosis	when the rapid heart rate is not an essential compensatory mechanism

With the exception of sotalol, beta blockers appear to have little place in the management of ventricular dysrhythmias.

CONTRAINDICATIONS

Should not be given to:

- patients whose heart rate is already slow
- patients with heart failure
- patients with cardiogenic shock
- concurrently with or within several days of discontinuing verapamil

Use with caution in the presence of:

- hypotension
- heart block
- chronic respiratory disease
- peripheral vascular disease
- diabetes

ADMINISTRATION

Oral

The undernoted doses are suggested for initial therapy and can be increased if necessary. Water-soluble beta blockers tend to be excreted unchanged by the kidneys, have longer half-lives and are often effective when taken only once daily.

acebutolol (Sectral) 100mg b.d.
atenolol (Tenormin) 50mg daily
metoprolol
(Betaloc, Lopresor) 50mg b.d.
nadolol (Corgard) 40mg daily
oxprenolol (Trasicor) 40mg b.d.
pindolol (Visken) 5mg b.d.

propranolol
(Berkolol, Inderal) 20mg b.d.
sotalol
(Beta-Cardone, Sotacor) 160mg daily
timolol
(Betim, Blocadren) 5mg b.d.

Long-acting preparations are expensive and though sometimes useful in the treatment of angina and hypertension are seldom required for disorders of rhythm.

Intravenous

Some beta blockers (acebutol, metoprolol, oxprenolol, propranolol, sotalol) can be used intravenously in emergencies that cannot be controlled by other means. They should only be given to patients who are under cardiological control.

SIDE EFFECTS

In the relatively small doses that are required to control disorders of rate and rhythm, beta blockers are usually well tolerated except in well-defined circumstances such as heart failure, bronchospasm and peripheral vascular disease.

Amongst side effects reported are:
- nausea, diarrhoea
- skin rashes, dry eyes
- insomnia, sleep disturbances, nightmares (less troublesome with the least lipid-soluble)
- weight gain
- paraesthesia
- lassitude, muscle fatigue and intermittent claudication
- coldness of extremities, especially in older patients (possibly less troublesome with those possessing partial agonist activity)

SUPERVISION AND FOLLOW UP

Patients on beta blockers are easily managed.

Note. Their dose is often reduced because they are found to have a slow heart rate. This should be ignored unless they also have symptoms suggesting that it is accompanied by an inadequate cardiac output.

Beta blockers should not be withdrawn suddenly in patients with coronary heart disease in case of rebound effects.

Cardiac Arrest

Cardiac arrest is said to have occurred if effective cardiac output suddenly ceases. It need not be asystolic, but can happen whenever the ventricular rate is either too fast or too slow to maintain an adequate circulation.

Causes
Commonest: ventricular fibrillation
Less often: ventricular asystole
Occasionally: very rapid ventricular tachycardia; very slow idioventricular rhythm

Occurrence
Usually:
- following acute myocardial infarction or an acute ischaemic episode in coronary heart disease
- during general anaesthesia
- as a terminal event in any severe organic disease

Also in:
- acute pulmonary disease
- drug poisoning
- electrocution
- drowning

Rarely: as a self-terminating event except in Adams-Stokes seizures.

CLINICAL FEATURES

Cardiac arrest is distinguished from other causes of sudden collapse by pulselessness. Absent breathing is usually also noticeable. Dilated pupils indicate cerebral anoxia.

ECG

The ECG reveals the causative rhythm. Most frequently, this is ventricular fibrillation (VF) or asystole. Occasionally, it is some other very rapid rhythm such as 1:1 flutter.

TREATMENT

Objectives
- to restore the circulation by cardiac compression
- to oxygenate the blood by artificial ventilation
- to correct acidosis with sodium bicarbonate
- to identify and terminate the causative rhythm

Procedures
Immediate:
- place the patient supine on a firm surface
- strike the lower sternum forcefully, once or twice

If ineffective:
- compress the heart by pressing downwards on the lower sternum approximately once a second
- another person must (i) establish an airway and (ii) start artificial respiration with:
  - the kiss of life
  - a face mask and bag
  - an endotracheal tube

As soon as possible:
- identify the rhythm when an ECG becomes available. If it is VF or a very rapid tachycardia, give a DC shock. If no ECG is available, assume that it is VF and give a shock.
- give IV sodium bicarbonate (1ml 8.4% per kg) and repeat after 10 minutes
- if asystole, give 10ml, 1:10,000 adrenaline and 10ml, 10% calcium chloride IV and insert a pacemaker if available

Cardioversion

Most serious disorders of rhythm can be terminated, at least temporarily, by giving the heart an electric shock through the chest wall. A direct current (DC) shock is best. It is usually timed to avoid the vulnerable part of the cardiac cycle and is delivered 0.02 seconds after the peak of the R wave on the ECG. It is very painful and distressing to conscious patients, so either make sure that they are unconscious or give a short-acting IV anaesthetic (10–30mg diazepam).

INDICATIONS

- to save life, as in ventricular fibrillation
- to terminate tachycardia, if it is resistant to drug therapy or causing rapid circulatory collapse
- to restore normal rhythm, if this does not occur spontaneously following treatment (e.g. in thyrotoxicosis or during cardiac surgery)

CONTRAINDICATIONS

Do not give a DC shock to fully digitalised patients or to patients whose disorders of rhythm might be caused by digitalis or quinidine, except in life-threatening emergencies.

TECHNIQUE

Smear both paddles liberally with electrode jelly. Place the electrodes:
- one in the right parasternal area
- one in the left axilla or below the left scapula

Charge the defibrillator to the desired level:
- 25–50 Watt seconds (Ws) for atrial flutter
- 100–400Ws for other tachycardias. Start at 100 and work up, giving a maximum of 4 or 5 shocks if unsuccessful.

Make certain that:
- the patient is unconscious
- no-one is touching the patient or the bed
- the ECG machine is temporarily switched off during the shock, unless it is suppressed

Discharge the electrode by pressing the button on the handle.
Reconnect the ECG machine immediately to observe the result.

SIDE EFFECTS AND COMPLICATIONS

To the patient
- slight skin burns are usually the only undesirable effect
- danger of serious dysrhythmia in fully digitalised patients
- risk of embolism in atrial fibrillation if not on anticoagulant therapy
- occasional pulmonary oedema has been reported

To the attendants: electrocution, if the paddles are not handled with care

To the equipment: upset by surge of electricity. Switch off, momentarily, if not specially adapted to withstand shocks.

SUPERVISION AND FOLLOW UP

Immediate postcardioversion period
Careful supervision under ECG control until:
- patient regains consciousness
- rhythm is stable
- complications have been excluded

Long-term follow up
Usually unnecessary unless:
- disorder recurs
- drug therapy is required to maintain normal rhythm

Digoxin
(Lanoxin)

ACTION

The principal therapeutic effects are mediated through increased vagal activity, which:
- enhances automaticity
- depresses conductivity in AV junctional tissues
- shortens the refractory period of atrial and ventricular myocardium

It also increases myocardial contractility.

Digoxin has complex, variable and sometimes paradoxical effects on different parts of the heart that, to some extent, depend upon its concentration in the tissues. IV digoxin acts within 15–30 minutes: maximum effect within 2 hours. Oral digoxin acts within 1–3 hours: maximum effect within 6–12 hours.

INDICATIONS

Digitalis is used to suppress or prevent:
- rapid supraventricular rhythms
- junctional ectopic rhythms

or where they cannot be suppressed, as in atrial fibrillation or atrial flutter, to slow the ventricular rate.

CONTRAINDICATIONS

Digoxin must *not* be used:
- if the abnormal rhythm might be due to digitalis toxicity, e.g. paroxysmal atrial tachycardia with block, bigeminal rhythm or ventricular tachycardia
- in hypertrophic obstructive cardiomyopathy

It should be used with caution in patients with heart block or hypokalaemia and in those who are on verapamil therapy.

Remember that DC shocks should not be given to patients who are fully digitalised or who have disorders caused by digitalis toxicity.

ADMINISTRATION

Orally
Initially: 0.5–1.0mg; followed by: 0.25–0.5mg daily.

Intravenously
0.5mg given very slowly. Use only in an emergency and only after confirming that the patient is not already on digitalis therapy.

Note. Elderly patients are often very sensitive to digitalis and require reduced (often paediatric) doses.

SIDE EFFECTS

- early toxic effects: anorexia, nausea
- later effects: vomiting, diarrhoea, headache, fatigue, malaise, insomnia, depression

ECG

- ventricular ectopic beats often occurring as coupled rhythm
- multifocal ectopic beats
- paroxysmal atrial tachycardia: especially in the elderly
- junctional tachycardia
- ventricular tachycardia: serious evidence of toxicity
- effects on conduction: may vary from lengthening of the PR interval to complete AV dissociation

Electrolyte imbalance

Disturbances of electrolyte balance induced by powerful diuretics, particularly potassium depletion, commonly precipitate disorders of rate, rhythm and conduction.

SUPERVISION AND FOLLOW UP

Patients taking digitalis require careful supervision, especially if they are elderly and also on diuretic therapy. Never ignore early warning symptoms of toxicity such as nausea and anorexia.

The ECG may be helpful in cases of doubt. It should seldom be necessary to assay the level of digoxin in the blood.

Disopyramide
(Dirythmin SA, Rythmodan)

ACTION

Disopyramide:
- decreases automaticity by delaying depolarisation
- increases the refractory period of atrial and ventricular myocardium by prolonging the duration of the action potential
- probably slows conduction in the His-Purkinje system

Like many drugs that act in this way, its effectiveness is decreased by hypokalaemia. Its half-life in normal subjects is 6–8 hours, but may be much longer in patients with heart disease.

INDICATIONS

Disopyramide is used to:
- control ectopic beats and tachycardias
- prevent ventricular dysrhythmias following myocardial infarction
- maintain sinus rhythm after cardioversion

CONTRAINDICATIONS

Disopyramide should not be given to patients who have:
- been taking other drugs that act in a similar manner or beta blockers
- hypotension
- untreated heart failure
- had too much digitalis
- 2nd or 3rd degree heart block
- sick sinus (tachycardia/bradycardia) syndrome
- impaired renal or hepatic function
- been receiving anticholinergic therapy
- hypokalaemia
- bundle branch block
- bradycardia that persists after treatment
- widening of the QRS complexes
- prolongation of the QT interval
- atrial flutter or paroxysmal atrial tachycardia

134

ADMINISTRATION

Orally
Initially: a loading dose of 300mg (omit if in doubt about possible contraindications); followed by 150mg every 6 hours; increasing to: 200mg if the desired effect is not achieved and there are no troublesome side effects.

Proportionally smaller doses should be used in patients weighing less than 50kg.

Intravenously
IV disopyramide should only be given in hospital and preferably in a coronary care unit with ECG monitoring.

Initially: a bolus of 2mg/kg (not exceeding 150mg) slowly over not less than 5 minutes; followed by 0.4mg/kg/hr (20–30mg); if necessary two additional half-strength boluses may be given.

The total dose should not exceed 300mg in 1 hour and 800mg in 24 hours.

SIDE EFFECTS

Effects due to anticholinergic action
- dry mouth
- blurred vision
- urinary retention
- glaucoma

Other side effects
- nausea, diarrhoea
- fatigue, muscle weakness
- dizziness

Occasionally reported
- heart failure
- acute psychoses
- cholestatic jaundice
- hypoglycaemia

Side effects usually disappear quickly when the dose is reduced or the drug is stopped.

SUPERVISION AND FOLLOW UP

Patients having intravenous infusion require constant ECG monitoring.

Patients on oral therapy require careful supervision. They should be advised to report any untoward effects immediately, because a reduced dose often minimises or abolishes them. They should be warned about the danger of taking drugs with a similar action or beta blockers while on treatment.

Isoprenaline
(Saventrine)

ACTION

Isoprenaline is a potent stimulator of beta adrenergic receptors with only a slight effect on alpha receptors. It is also a powerful cardiac stimulant with both chronotropic and inotropic actions. In addition it:
- stimulates all cardiac pacemakers
- increases myocardial contractility
- causes peripheral vasodilatation

INDICATIONS

It is effective in maintaining heart rate and cardiac output in high grade heart block occurring spontaneously or following myocardial infarction.

Recently, it has been largely superseded by safe and reliable cardiac pacemakers, but is still used in extreme bradycardia or asystole until a pacemaker is inserted and functioning satisfactorily.

CONTRAINDICATIONS

Isoprenaline should be given with caution, especially if used intravenously in:
- acute myocardial infarction
- heart failure
- cardiogenic shock

In these circumstances, it increases the oxygen demand of the already compromised myocardium and is liable to cause ventricular tachycardia or ventricular fibrillation, so it is better to use atropine for severe bradycardia.

ADMINISTRATION

Intravenously
Initially: a bolus of 0.1mg isoprenaline hydrochloride; followed by an infusion (100 drops per minute) of 2mg in 500ml of 5% laevulose.

Orally
Initially: one 30mg tablet, three times daily; increasing to several times this dose until:
- the optimum effect is achieved
- side effects restrict its usefulness

SIDE EFFECTS

- flushing, sweats, tremor
- palpitations, precordial distress
- headaches
- diarrhoea

SUPERVISION AND FOLLOW UP

Intravenous therapy is hazardous and should only be used under strict cardiological control.

Oral therapy is less dangerous, but elderly patients require careful supervision to ensure that the drug is achieving the desired effect without causing too much upset.

Lignocaine
(Xylocard)

ACTION

Lignocaine's main action is in the ventricles where it:
- decreases excitability
- depresses intraventricular conduction velocity
- reduces the maximal rate of stimulation to which they can respond
- abolishes repetitive responses to single premature beats

and also in the His-Purkinje system where it:
- depresses automaticity
- prolongs the refractory period
- raises the threshold to stimulation

Lignocaine:
- has no effect on the SA node
- little effect on other supraventricular tissues
- causes minimal prolongation of AV conduction time

It is therefore of little use in supraventricular dysrhythmias.
    Its half-life in normal subjects is about two hours.

INDICATIONS

The prevention and suppression of ventricular dysrhythmias following acute myocardial infarction.

CONTRAINDICATIONS

Lignocaine should *not* be used in patients who:
- are hypersensitive to local anaesthetics of the amide type
- have second or third degree heart block, as it reduces the automaticity of ventricular pacemakers

It should be used *with caution* in the presence of:
- lesser degrees of heart block
- bradycardia
- hypotension
- heart failure

ADMINISTRATION

Intravenous infusion
Initially: a bolus of 100mg over 2 minutes; followed by 2mg per minute for 36 hours. If necessary, give two further boluses and increase the infusion rate to 4mg per minute (maximum).

In shock, severe heart failure, grossly impaired hepatic or renal function, reduce the dose by 50%.

Intramuscularly
300mg to patients with recent myocardial infarction during transit to CCU.

SIDE EFFECTS

Cardiovascular
- bradycardia
- hypotension
- prolongation of PR interval, widening of QRS complex
- cardiac arrest

Central nervous system
- nausea, cold sweats
- pallor, tremor
- respiratory depression
- drowsiness, disorientation
- agitation, euphoria
- tremor, blurred vision
- convulsions, coma

SUPERVISION AND FOLLOW UP

Patients on lignocaine infusions require careful monitoring under constant ECG control. As therapy is of relatively short duration and can only be given intravenously, it should be followed by an oral preparation with similar properties, e.g. tocainide, mexiletine or disopyramide.

Mexiletine
(Mexitil)

ADMINISTRATION

Orally
Initially: a loading dose of 400mg; followed after two hours by 200–300mg three times daily.

Intravenously
In acute situations this requires careful clinical and ECG control in coronary care units.

Initially: a bolus of 150mg is given slowly over 5–10 minutes; followed by 250mg in the first hour, 500mg over the next 8 hours and 500mg over the next 12 hours.

If necessary, two additional boluses of 50mg may be given.

ACTION

Mexiletine is structurally similar to lignocaine and acts in a similar way. It delays depolarisation and decreases automaticity in the ventricles, without greatly affecting the resting potential or prolonging the action potential. It also has little effect on supraventricular tissues. Its half-life in normal subjects is 9–12 hours, but may be much longer in patients with heart disease.

INDICATIONS

It is used to prevent and suppress ventricular dysrhythmias, particularly those following myocardial infarction. It has the advantage over lignocaine that it can be given by mouth, but the disadvantage that it is much more likely to cause troublesome side effects.

CONTRAINDICATIONS

Give with caution to patients with:
- hypotension
- severe heart failure
- sinus node dysfunction
- high grade heart block
- renal or hepatic failure
- Parkinsonism

SIDE EFFECTS

Gastro-intestinal
- nausea, indigestion
- vomiting, diarrhoea

Cardiovascular
- hypotension
- bradycardia
- atrial fibrillation

Central nervous system (common)
- lightheadedness, dizziness
- confusion, drowsiness, dysarthia
- blurred vision, diplopia, nystagmus
- paraesthesia, tremor, ataxia
- convulsions

SUPERVISION AND FOLLOW UP

Careful supervision is required because of side effects, many of which can be most unpleasant. These are, however, closely related to blood levels and can often be minimised or made tolerable by reducing the dose, without abolishing the beneficial effects.

Pacing

If necessary, the electromechanical activity of the heart can be controlled with one of the many increasingly sophisticated types of pacemaker that are now becoming available.

Pacing is usually carried out by passing an electrode-tipped catheter from a peripheral vein into the heart. The catheter is attached to a battery-operated power supply that transmits current to the electrode. The myocardium contracts each time the electrode discharges.

Pacemakers are either temporary or permanent

With temporary pacemakers, the power source is contained in a box outside the body and the controls can easily be manipulated to suit the circumstances.

With permanent pacemakers, the power source and the controls have to be implanted, usually in the pectoral region. As they have to be programmed before insertion, they are necessarily less adaptable than temporary pacemakers, although some of the newer models can be adjusted without having to expose them surgically.

Types of pacemakers

Most pacemakers in current use are of the on-demand ventricular type that come into action if the spontaneous rate falls below 70 per minute. They are relatively cheap and trouble free, but are unphysiological in that the synchrony between atrial and ventricular contraction is lost and the heart rate cannot respond to the needs of the patient.

Several types of more complicated pacemakers are now on the market that can pace both chambers, or pace one having sensed the other. They are not yet trouble free and though still expensive, clearly point the way ahead.

Identification of pacemakers

Pacemakers can be identified by a code that uses the following letters:
A = atrium: V = ventricle: D = atrium and ventricle:
I = inhibited: T = triggered: O = not applicable

To interpret the code:
- the first letter indicates the chamber that is being paced
- the second letter indicates the chamber whose activity is sensed
- the third letter indicates the response of the pacemaker to sensing, i.e. whether it is being inhibited or triggered by spontaneous heart action

Example 1
On-demand ventricular pacing = VVI. (The pacing electrode is in the ventricle. The sensing electrode is also in the ventricle and inhibits the pacemaker unless spontaneous activation falls below a given rate.)

Example 2
Atrial synchronous pacing = VAT. (The pacing electrode is in the ventricle. The sensing electrode is in the atrium and triggers the ventricular pacemaker when it detects atrial activation.)

INDICATIONS

Temporary pacing

This is most frequently required following acute myocardial infarction in patients who develop, or are thought likely to develop, high grade heart block.

It is occasionally necessary:
- in poisoning with digitalis or beta blockers
- in the acute phase of such diseases as
  - myocarditis
  - sarcoidosis
  - amyloidosis
  - collagenosis
- during or after cardiac surgery
- to control rapid rhythms that are resistant to drug therapy

Permanent pacing

This is most frequently required by patients with complete heart block or the sick sinus syndrome whose heart rate is too slow to maintain an adequate circulation, or who are having giddy turns or Adams Stokes attacks.

It is sometimes required:
- following myocardial infarction
- as a result of cardiac surgery
- in congenital heart block
- to control disorders of rate, rhythm or conduction

COMPLICATIONS

Complications should not be troublesome nowadays. When present, they may be related to the pulse generator:
- haematoma
- sepsis
- stimulation of the pectoral tissues

Alternatively, they may affect the pacing electrode:
- dislocation
- exit block
- failure to sense
- stimulation of the diaphragm

Any of these may necessitate re-implantation of the generator or repositioning (replacement) of the catheter.

SUPERVISION AND FOLLOW UP

Temporary pacemakers

Patients with temporary pacemakers require constant short-term supervision and should be under cardiological control throughout the procedure.

Permanent pacemakers

Patients with permanent pacemakers can lead normal or near-normal lives, but should be seen regularly (every six months) by skilled technicians at a cardiac clinic where the system can be checked over and pacemaker failure detected or anticipated.

Modern pacemakers have lithium batteries with a minimum life of four years and a maximum life of fifteen years; so power failure is nothing like the problem it used to be.

Electromagnetic interference from outside sources, which used to inhibit pacemakers, has been largely overcome, though patients should avoid microwave ovens and high voltage circuits. Defibrillation may damage pacemakers if the paddles are not kept well away from them during DC cardioversion. Diathermy may temporarily inhibit them and surgeons need to be aware of this danger.

Driving

An ordinary driving licence may be held if a pacemaker has been functioning satisfactorily for at least three months and the patient regularly attends a pacemaker clinic. The Licencing Centre should be notified. Patients with pacemakers may *not* hold HGV or PSV licences.

Death

The clinic should be informed immediately a patient dies, so that the pacemaker can be removed before burial or cremation.

Phenytoin Sodium
(Epanutin)

ACTION

Phenytoin, well known for its control of epilepsy, decreases AV conduction time and suppresses ectopic beats. It also impairs myocardial contractility.

INDICATIONS

A little-used antidysrhythmic drug that is of value in the treatment of dysrhythmias caused by digitalis toxicity. It should only be used in emergencies under continuous ECG control where cardiac resuscitation is readily available. In the treatment of other abnormalities it is less effective than alternative drugs currently available.

CONTRAINDICATIONS

Care is required with intravenous use. Phenytoin depresses cardiac function, particularly in:
- the elderly
- patients with heart failure

It should not be used in the presence of:
- hypotension
- severe bradycardia
- high grade heart block

Warnings
- Phenytoin is highly alkaline and incompatible with all other solutions. It must be given alone and should *not* be added to other infusions.
- Subcutaneous and perivascular injection cause tissue damage.
- Several drugs, including dicourmarol anticoagulants, have been shown to elevate phenytoin plasma levels.

ADMINISTRATION

Phenytoin therapy requires careful control and should be reserved for the short-term hospital treatment of patients whose abnormal rhythm is the result of overdosage with digitalis. It is absorbed slowly when given by mouth; maximum plasma levels are only reached after 8–12 hours.

145

Intravenous therapy
3.5–5mg/kg by slow infusion not exceeding 50mg per minute. This may be repeated once if necessary. If given quickly, it is likely to cause bradycardia and hypotension.

If successful, change to oral therapy: 200–250mg b.d.

SIDE EFFECTS

Many side effects have been reported, including ventricular fibrillation, asystolic arrest and tonic seizures.

Procainamide
(Pronestyl)

ACTION

Procainamide:
- reduces myocardial excitability, conductivity and contractility
- depresses automaticity in the His-Purkinje system
- increases the refractory period of the atrial and ventricular myocardium

Its half-life in normal subjects is 3–5 hours.

INDICATIONS

It is effective in the prevention and suppression of supraventricular, junctional and ventricular dysrhythmias.

CONTRAINDICATIONS

It should not be given to patients who are:
- hypotensive, because it often aggravates the condition
- in high grade heart block, because it depresses ventricular automaticity

It should be given with caution to patients with:
- bundle branch block

It is not recommended for patients with:
- asthma
- a history of allergy
- atrial fibrillation or flutter, because it may increase the ventricular rate

ADMINISTRATION

Orally
Initially: a loading dose of 500–1000mg; followed by 250–500mg every 4–6 hours. Using a long-acting preparation a loading dose of 1.5–2.0g; followed by 1.0–1.5g three times daily.

Intravenously
- highly effective
- extremely dangerous
- should only be given under cardiological control

147

An initial dose of 100mg in dilute solution is given very slowly (over several minutes). This can be repeated, but under no circumstances should the total dose exceed 1.0g.

The ECG and blood pressure should be monitored carefully throughout the injection, which should be stopped immediately if the:

- desired effect is achieved
- blood pressure falls
- PR interval becomes prolonged
- QRS complex widens

SIDE EFFECTS

Procainamide is usually well tolerated, but a wide variety of side effects have been reported:

- anorexia, nausea, vomiting, diarrhoea
- pruritis, skin rashes
- allergic reactions, leucopenia
- chills, fever, flushing
- vertigo, dizziness, headache
- hallucinations
- lupus erythematosis-like syndrome

SUPERVISION AND FOLLOW UP

Procainamide is a useful and effective antidysrhythmic agent but the LE-like syndrome has restricted its use to short-term therapy, because it does not always go away when treatment is discontinued.

It should not normally be given for more than six weeks. If long-term suppressive therapy is required, it should be replaced by some other drug with a similar mode of action.

Psychosomatic Therapy

The heart is extremely sensitive to psychic stimuli. Both the sympathetic and parasympathetic nerves, as well as the thyroid and adrenal glands, can exert profound influences on the cardiovascular system in normal people as well as in those with heart disease.

Some are much more sensitive than others in this regard; not only on the effect that mind has over matter, but in their reaction to it. Having become aware of their heart, they are conscious of and worried by every ectopic beat. In contrast, others appear completely unaware of it, even during a paroxysm when the heart is pounding, and throbbing can be seen in the root of the neck.

These behaviour patterns have an important bearing on the management of patients, because it is never a good thing to focus attention on things that do not trouble them or about which they do not complain.

Personality patterns, life styles and reactions to them, are factors that may cause or influence disorders of rate, rhythm and conduction. These may typically be:

- chronic anxiety
- excessive hostility
- constant frustration
- compulsive behaviour
- worry and depression

Circumstances that might exacerbate the problem should always be sought for and discussed. For example:

- fear
- anger
- undue excitement
- excessive fatigue
- lack of sleep
- unhappy love affairs
- danger
- bereavement

Patients under these kinds of stresses often:

- smoke too many cigarettes
- drink too much tea, coffee, alcohol

Remember too, that many patients with heart disease, or who think that they have heart disease, live with the constant and secret fear of dropping down dead. In these circumstances, consciousness of an abnormal heart beat often sets up a vicious circle that is difficult to break.

In some cases, a simple explanation about the power of psyche over soma, coupled with a sympathetic attitude, is all that is required. In others, more strenuous and continued effort is required, together with the use of sedative or antidysrhythmic drugs, or both.

149

Quinidine Bisulphate
(Kinidin)

ACTION

Quinidine:
- depresses automaticity, excitability and conductivity, and prolongs the refractory period in the atria
- depresses automaticity, slows conduction and prolongs the refractory period in the His-Purkinje system
- depresses excitability and conductivity in the ventricles
- has little or no effect on conduction through the AV node, although in some it may be enhanced

These effects are more pronounced when the heart rate is rapid than when it is relatively slow.

It also affects myocardial contractility, particularly:
- in the elderly
- in those with organic heart disease
- where the circulatory state has already deteriorated because of the dysrhythmia

Its half-life is about seven hours.

INDICATIONS

Quinidine can:
- suppress and prevent atrial, junctional and ventricular ectopic beats and tachycardias
- restore and maintain normal sinus rhythm in patients with atrial fibrillation and flutter, but if sinus rhythm is not restored, digoxin is preferable because it slows the ventricular rate

CONTRAINDICATIONS

It should not be given to patients with:
- a history of drug sensitivity
- heart block
- severe hypotension
- atrial flutter who are not digitalised. Alone it may increase the ventricular rate (danger of 1:1 flutter).

It should be given with caution in the presence of:
- heart failure
- digitalis toxicity
- hyperkalaemia

ADMINISTRATION

Oral therapy
Initially 200mg to test for sensitivity; followed by 200–300mg four to six times daily.
    Alternatively, using a long-acting preparation: 500–1250mg twice daily.

SIDE EFFECTS

Hypersensitivity
- urticaria
- pyrexia
- thrombocytopenia

Gastro-intestinal
- nausea
- vomiting
- diarrhoea

Cerebral
- blurred vision
- hearing disturbances
- headache and dizziness

Cardiovascular
- hypotension
- aggravation of heart failure
- serious dysrhythmias

ECG (early)
- prolongation of QT interval
- decrease in amplitude of T waves
- depression of ST segments

ECG (late)
- widening of QRS

SUPERVISION AND FOLLOW UP

Patients on maintenance therapy require regular surveillance. Careful clinical examination, ECGs and determination of plasma quinidine levels should prevent the development of serious toxicity.

Tocainide
(Tonocard)

ACTION

Tocainide has similar electrophysiological actions to lignocaine. Its half-life is 11–15 hours.

INDICATIONS

The prevention and suppression of acute and chronic ventricular dysrhythmias.

CONTRAINDICATIONS

It should *not* be used in patients who:
- are sensitive to amide drugs
- have high grade heart block

It should be used with caution in:
- bradycardia
- hypotension
- heart failure
- hepatic or renal disease
- the elderly
- those having other antidysrhythmic drugs

ADMINISTRATION

Orally
- 600mg b.d.
- may be increased to a maximum of twice this dose if necessary

Intravenously
- a slow infusion of 500–750mg, followed by:
- 600–800mg by mouth and then maintenance oral therapy

Bradycardia and hypotension may occur after IV injection.

In heart failure or in grossly impaired hepatic or renal function, the dose should be reduced by 50%.

SIDE EFFECTS

Hypersensitivity
- skin rashes
- fever
- transient neutropenia

Gastro-intestinal
- anorexia
- nausea
- vomiting
- abdominal pain
- constipation

Cerebral
- tremor
- dizziness
- convulsions
- paraesthesia

Rarely
- LE-like syndrome
- fibrosing alveolitis
- agranulocytosis

SUPERVISION AND FOLLOW UP

Care is required with long-term therapy. Side effects are mostly related to peak plasma concentrations and are therefore dose-related.

The rarer serious side effects demand immediate withdrawal of therapy.

Vagal Stimulation

Vagal stimulation is often helpful in diagnosis and sometimes in therapy.

The SA and AV nodes are supplied by both vagal nerves, but the main contribution to the SA node is from the right vagus and the main contribution to the AV node is from the left vagus.

Stimulation of the vagus releases acetylcholine and this:
- slows the heart rate
- increases the degree of AV block
- may even cause ventricular standstill

METHODS OF APPLICATION

Carotid sinus pressure activates the stretch receptors and causes reflex stimulation of the vagal and inhibition of the sympathetic nerves. This is the method most commonly used by clinicians. External pressure is applied gently on one side at a time; never on both sides together.

Some people are extremely sensitive to this test, which may result in profound bradycardia and hypotension. In elderly patients it may cause cerebral ischaemia.

The Valsalva manoeuvre is forced expiration against a closed glottis following deep inspiration. It increases the intrapleural pressure and initiates a vagal reflex by stimulating stretch receptors in the lungs.

The Müller procedure is forced inspiration against a closed glottis following deep expiration.

Other methods

Holding the breath in deep inspiration for as long as possible and then suddenly releasing it.

A finger or spoon handle pressed on the back of the tongue to induce gagging or retching.

An ice-collar placed around the neck.

Immersing the face in cold water.

Eyeball pressure, though often highly effective, is *not* recommended because it is extremely unpleasant and painful when carried out properly, and it may also damage the retina.

DIAGNOSIS

Vagal stimulation has an important role in the diagnosis of tachycardias and should always be tried before other methods are used or therapy is started.

As it also has a therapeutic effect in some cases, it should always be carried out under ECG control, if this is possible, so that a correct diagnosis can be made.

Sinus tachycardia: usually has no effect, but may occasionally cause slight slowing while the stimulus is applied.

Paroxysmal supraventricular and junctional tachycardia: either stops the paroxysm or has no effect on it.

Atrial tachycardia with AV block: often causes transient slowing of the ventricular rate by increasing the degree of AV block.

Atrial flutter: may slow the ventricular rate and reveal the flutter waves by temporarily increasing the degree of AV block.

Atrial fibrillation: usually has no appreciable effect, but may slow ventricular rate a little.

Ventricular tachycardia: has no effect.

TREATMENT

Vagal stimulation has limited therapeutic value, because in so many cases it only affects the rate and rhythm while the stimulus is being applied.

In some patients with paroxysmal tachycardia, however, it is highly effective. If this is found to be the case, it is well worth while teaching them how to terminate a paroxysm using one or other of the methods noted above.

Verapamil
(Cordilox)

ACTION

Verapamil is a calcium antagonist that has a powerful depressant effect on the AV node. It:
- lengthens the refractory period
- increases transnodal conduction time

It also depresses the discharge rate from the SA node.
Its half-life in normal subjects is three to seven hours.

INDICATIONS

Verapamil is highly effective in terminating paroxysmal supraventricular tachycardia of the re-entrant type when given intravenously. Oral therapy, though less effective, may be of benefit in selected cases.

CONTRAINDICATIONS

Verapamil should *not* be given to patients who are taking or who have recently been taking beta blockers or digitalis, in whom it may cause:
- severe bradycardia
- profound hypotension
- heart block
- asystolic arrest

Neither should it be given to patients who have:
- hypotension
- high grade heart block
- heart failure
- cardiac shock

Nor to patients with the sick sinus (tachycardia/bradycardia) syndrome

Verapamil should be used with caution in:
- the acute phase of myocardial infarction
- patients with impaired liver function

156

ADMINISTRATION

Intravenously
- 5mg by slow injection. This may be repeated once or twice after 5–10 minutes if necessary.
- 5–10mg by infusion over 1 hour with a maximum of 100mg in 24 hours

Verapamil should only be used intravenously in hospital under ECG control.

Orally
40mg t.d.s. This may be doubled or trebled if necessary.

SIDE EFFECTS

The following occur occasionally after IV use:
- severe hypotension
- heart block
- ventricular fibrillation
- asystole

Oral verapamil is generally well tolerated. Nausea, vomiting, constipation, flushing and dizziness have been reported.

SUPERVISION AND FOLLOW UP

Patients receiving Verapamil require regular supervison. If it is not effective, it should be stopped before other drugs that depress myocardial function are prescribed, because of its additive effects.

6

PATIENT-MANAGEMENT PROBLEMS

The following fictitious problems have been devised to illustrate how to recognise presenting features, decide which disorder is likely to be causing them, and prescribe appropriate treatment.

Although constructed around general practitioners, hospital doctors and nurses, all will be of value to anyone who wishes to learn more about disorders of rate, rhythm and conduction. Each contains extensive cross references to appropriate sections in the book to help resolve any difficulties that may arise while working through them.

GENERAL PRACTITIONER PROBLEMS

A Young Man with Palpitation

William Stark, aged 37, is a sales manager with a car firm. His wife works as a part-time staff nurse in the coronary care unit at the local hospital. She had phoned in the afternoon to make an appointment for him to be seen at the evening surgery.

He tells you that he has had attacks of palpitation during the past four weeks. They have been decreasing in frequency and he had only told his wife about them earlier that day. He has no history suggestive of heart disease. He had a 'flu'-like illness about five weeks ago. He smokes at least twenty cigarettes a day and drinks about ten cups of black coffee. He is a social drinker.

What questions would you ask Mr. Stark?

You ask:	*Mr. Stark answers:*
What do you mean by palpitation?	I feel a thumping in my chest.
During an attack, is it there all the time or does it come and go?	It is constant.
How does it start?	It starts abruptly.
How long does it last?	It usually lasts about twenty minutes, sometimes less, sometimes more.
How often does it occur?	It has been happening a lot less in the last few days, but say about two or three times in a day.
How fast is the heart beat during attacks? Tap it on your hand.	(It is about 140 per minute.)
How does it stop?	It stops as abruptly as it started. One moment it is there; the next moment it has gone.

What conclusion should you draw from this history?

- that he is having paroxysmal tachycardia

What further information would help to determine the nature of the paroxysmal tachycardia?

You ask:	*Mr. Stark answers:*
Mr. Stark, is the thumping regular or irregular?	The thumping is regular.

In this case, the patient says that the 'thumping' is regular. However, it must be kept in mind that at rates above 160 per minute it becomes increasingly difficult to differentiate between regular and irregular palpitation. Irregular beating suggests atrial fibrillation.

(See page 35 for more about the symptoms of palpitation and how to take a history from a patient with this complaint.)

What is the most likely diagnosis and what is your differential diagnosis?

- paroxysmal supraventricular or junctional tachycardia is far and away the most likely cause of his palpitation
- paroxysmal ventricular tachycardia is not likely in the absence of serious heart disease, although it is occasionally seen in apparently healthy people
- paroxysmal atrial flutter, in the absence of serious heart disease or as a lone condition, is also uncommon at this age
- atrial tachycardia with AV block is also most unlikely in a person of this age, especially in someone not taking digoxin

(These abnormal rhythms are described and illustrated on: pages 52, 68, 77, 62 and 56.)

You now examine the patient. What would you expect to find?

- the pulse rate is 80 per minute and regular
- physical examination reveals no abnormality
- the blood pressure is 125/85mm Hg

What points in the history might help you to explain why he is getting palpitation?

- a week before the palpitation began he had a viral illness that may have affected his myocardium
- he smokes 20 cigarettes a day. This may have exacerbated the condition
- he drinks ten cups of coffee a day. Caffeine may also be an aetiological factor.

(See page 52 for the aetiology of supraventricular tachycardia.)

What is your provisional diagnosis?

- he has paroxysmal supraventricular tachycardia, possibly caused by a virus infection and aggravated by smoking and by drinking too much coffee

What further investigations would you carry out?

- no further investigations are necessary. For example, it is much too late to carry out viral studies, but on principle, a 12 lead ECG should be recorded.

While you are seeing the next patient, your practice nurse takes the following ECG.

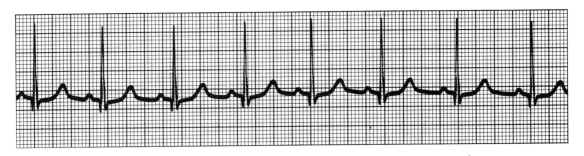

How do you interpret it?

- it shows normal sinus rhythm

(Normal sinus rhythm: see page 39.)

Having seen the ECG, you see Mr. Stark and his wife in your consulting room.

How would you manage things from here?

- allow the couple to ventilate their fears about what the diagnosis might have been
- communicate your findings to the patient and his wife
- explain that the condition is not serious, pointing out that it is already becoming less troublesome daily and that you are sure it will go away without doing any permanent damage to the heart. Tell them also that no drug treatment is necessary.
- advise him to give up smoking and cut down on his coffee drinking

The fact that Mrs. Stark made the appointment when she found out about his palpitation, despite the fact that Mr. Stark admitted things were improving, indicates her anxiety. The knowledge that she works in a coronary care unit must be kept in mind when reassuring her.

(Therapeutic principles: see page 119. Specific treatment: see page 54.)

Despite your reassurance, Mrs. Stark arranges for a 24-hour tape recording to be done on her husband, at the hospital. An excerpt is shown here.

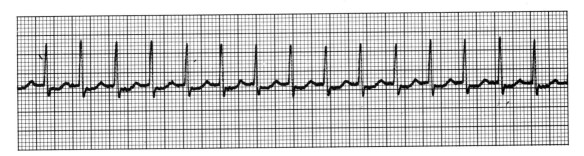

What does it show?

- supraventricular tachycardia

SUMMARY

This was a problem about paroxysmal supraventricular tachycardia occurring in a healthy young man. It illustrates that this is not necessarily a serious condition and that it often disappears spontaneously. In these circumstances, no specific treatment is required other than an explanation and reassurance.

Sudden Illness on the Golf Course

Sandy MacPherson is a 53 year-old engineer who became ill while playing on the local golf course. He described the sudden onset of a rapid heart beat. This was associated with breathlessness and a feeling of fatigue. He rested over his golf bag and then sat down for a little while, but the palpitation persisted and, as he felt unwell, he called it a day and drove home.

His wife contacts you as it is your evening 'on call'. She is clearly concerned because he has never had a day's illness in his life. In response to a question, she tells you that he has had no chest pain.

What would you do about it?

* you should go at once

The sudden onset of tachycardia severe enough to cause symptoms in a previously healthy patient of this age must always be taken seriously. He may have had a coronary heart attack.

When you arrive he is sitting up in bed, ashen-grey, breathless and sweating a little. His heart rate is 160 per minute. His blood pressure is 100/60. He has some fine crepitations at both lung bases.

What further history would you take?

You ask:	*Mr. MacPherson answers:*
Has the rapid beating been constantly present since it started suddenly on the golf course?	Yes; it has been going on ever since I drove off at the 11th tee more than two hours ago.
Has the rate changed at all?	No, it has been steady like this.
Has it felt regular or irregular?	It has been regular throughout.
Have you ever had anything like this before?	No, never.
You say you have had no pain: have you any other feeling in your chest?	A slight tightness across my upper chest. Oh, and a numb, heavy feeling in my left arm; I thought I might have strained it driving.
Ever had any tightness before?	No, never.
Any family history of heart trouble?	My father died of a coronary when he was 66.
What about smoking?	At least 30 cigarettes every day.

(The information required to help assess the nature and severity of such attacks is given on pages 34–38.)

What conclusion do you draw from this history?

- he has a paroxysm of tachycardia that may well be associated with acute myocardial ischaemia

If it is, what is the likely nature of the paroxysm?

- it is likely to be ventricular in origin

What would you do next?

- you should record an ECG

The bizarre nature of the QRS complexes makes interpretation difficult, but a rhythm strip (seen below) indicates the nature of the paroxysm.

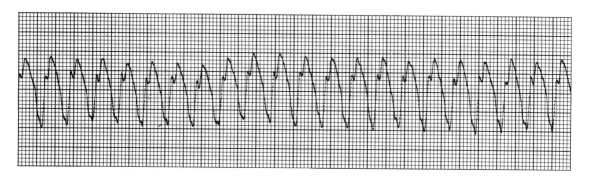

What does it show?

- it shows ventricular tachycardia

(Ventricular tachycardia: see page 77.)

What management would you recommend?

- he should be moved to hospital immediately. Preferably after treatment by a mobile coronary care unit, or at least in an ambulance with facilities for resuscitation.

While you are waiting for transport what measures would you take?

- give lignocaine 100mg intravenously, as a bolus injection, slowly, over two minutes
- monitor his pulse carefully
- explain to the patient and his wife what you think has happened and why he has to be sent to hospital

(The treatment of ventricular tachycardia: see page 79. Lignocaine therapy: see page 138.)

While you are waiting for help to arrive, the pulse disappears and the following ECG is recorded.

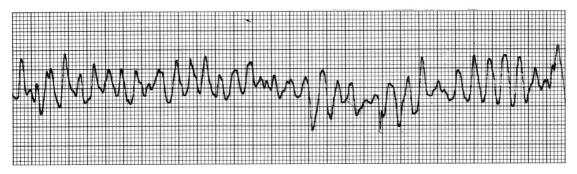

What does it show?

- that he has developed ventricular fibrillation

(Ventricular fibrillation: see page 80.)

What action would you take?

- move the patient onto the floor
- remove any false teeth
- give him a powerful thump over the lower sternum
- commence external cardiac massage
- ask his wife, or anyone else handy, to commence mouth-to-mouth respiration

After ten minutes of attempted resuscitation, he shows no sign of recovery and his ECG shows asystole.

(The treatment of cardiac arrest: see page 128. Asystole: see page 82.)

What would you do?

- decide that the patient was dead and that further attempts at resuscitation were unlikely to succeed
- inform Mrs. MacPherson that her husband was dead
- deal with the immediate effects of bereavement on the family
- issue a death certificate and inform her that she should contact the funeral directors

SUMMARY

This was a problem about the onset of tachycardia in a middle-aged man in circumstances that suggested the possibility of an acute coronary heart attack. It illustrates the serious nature of such a complication. Rapid ventricular rhythms demand urgent attention and are the most frequent cause of sudden death.

165

An Anxious Elderly Spinster

Audrey Fitzpatrick, a 73 year-old spinster, is a retired civil servant who lives with a widowed sister. They are well known to you as patients, having had many consultations over a number of years for a variety of symptoms that you have classified as anxiety neurosis. Both are on nightly sedation. Miss Fitzpatrick also has hypertension for which you have prescribed 5mg bendrofluazide each morning.

She comes, with her sister, to see you on a Saturday morning, complaining of 'utter exhaustion' associated with 'dreadful palpitation' for the last two weeks.

What further history would you take to elucidate the nature of her symptoms?

You ask:	Miss Fitzpatrick answers:
What do you mean by palpitation?	I can feel my heart beating.
What do you feel?	A strange sensation behind my breastbone. It appears to miss beats and to give very powerful beats.
How often do you get it?	On and off, all day long. Sometimes I think it has gone and then it starts again with a thump.
Is it troublesome at any special time?	It is usually worst when I am sitting quietly or lying in bed and is less troublesome when I am busy.
How fast is your heart beating when you have this palpitation? Could you tap it out for me?	(She taps a rate of 70–80 per minute minute on the table top.)
Is it regular or irregular?	It seems quite irregular. During a bad bad attack my heart feels quite higgledy-piggledy.

(An account of palpitation and the information necessary to assess its significance is given on page 35.)

After hearing this story, what do you think is the likely cause of her symptoms?

- the history suggests that the palpitation is due to ectopic beats

What would you do next?

You should continue the history to find out if:
- there is any obvious cause for the sudden onset of her symptoms two weeks ago
- she has ever had anything like this before
- the dysrhythmia is causing any haemodynamic upset

What questions would you ask?

You ask:	*Miss Fitzpatrick answers:*
Do you smoke?	No. I never have.
Do you drink tea?	Yes, but only a normal amount.
Do you drink coffee?	Only an occasional cup.
Do you drink alcohol?	I am a teetotaller.
Have you been taking any medicines?	No.
Have you had any recent infective illness?	No.
Have you been upset emotionally about anything recently?	Yes. I have been upset by the sudden death of my brother. I was devoted to him.
Do you know why he died?	They say it was his heart.
Have you had any symptoms that have made you think that you may have heart disease?	No, not that I know of.
What about the 'utter exhaustion'?	Oh, that is not unusual, I often find that I do too much and get very tired.
Have you ever before had anything like this palpitation?	Occasionally, on and off over the years, but never anything like so bad as this.
What happened in previous attacks?	They just gradually wore off.

(Atrial ectopic beats: see page 49. Ventricular ectopic beats: see page 73.)

What would you do next?

- you should examine her cardiovascular system and record an ECG

The examination reveals the following:

pulse: 80 per minute and occasionally irregular
blood pressure: 200/110
heart:
- the heart sounds are irregular with extra sounds and long, compensatory pauses
- no murmurs are heard
- the heart is slightly enlarged

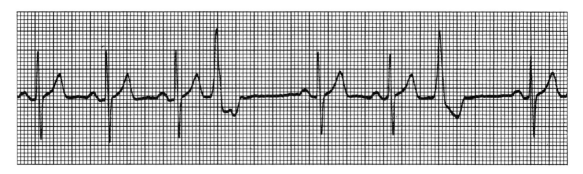

What conclusions would you make from these findings?

• that her symptoms are due to multiple ventricular ectopic beats

What is their significance?

• although ventricular ectopic beats are much less common than supraventricular ectopic beats, they do not necessarily have any significance; especially in a patient of this age with long-standing hypertension

What would you do about it?

• you should explain the nature of the palpitations to Miss Fitzpatrick, and to her sister, emphasising that there is nothing to worry about
• you should tell them that the attacks will probably wear off as they have on previous occasions and that no treatment is required

If they do not wear off and she comes back demanding treatment, what would you prescribe?

• a choice of drugs is available. In alphabetical order they are: disopyramide, mexiletine, procainamide, quinidine and sotalol. None is ideal and all have potentially unpleasant side effects, but sotalol might be tried in the first instance.

(The treatment of ventricular ectopic beats: see page 76. Specific drug therapy is detailed as follows: disopyramide, page 134; mexiletine, page 140; procainamide, page 147; quinidine, page 150; sotalol, page 125.)

SUMMARY

This was a problem about ectopic beats in an elderly patient who was already inclined to take her symptoms rather too seriously. It illustrates that even when they are ventricular in origin, they do not necessarily have any ominous significance and usually require no specific therapy.

Heart Failure and Weight Loss in Middle Age

Vicki Gibson is 48 years-old. Her husband is a wealthy business executive and they have always enjoyed a fairly extravagant life-style.

She comes complaining of tiredness and breathlessness and that she has been losing weight. She has smoked heavily for many years and her recurrent cough has recently become much more troublesome, especially when she is hurrying and when she lies down in bed at night. The cough is unproductive and she has had no haemoptysis.

During the last few months she has become increasingly aware of palpitation, usually when she is coughing or exerting herself, but sometimes for no apparent reason.

What possible causes of these symptoms are running through your mind?

- loss of weight in a heavy smoker of this age, associated with increased respiratory symptoms, should always suggest the possibility of a bronchial carcinoma
- on the other hand, certain of her symptoms suggest that she might have incipient left heart failure

Which of her symptoms suggest heart failure?

- a dry, irritating, unproductive cough that occurs on exertion and when she lies down in bed at night

What further information would you seek to amplify this part of her history?

You ask:	*Mrs. Gibson answers:*
Have you ever been wakened during the night by breathlessness?	Yes, occasionally, after a particularly busy day.
What happened?	I had to sit up in bed till it wore off Once, I had to get up and go to the window for air.
How many pillows do you sleep with?	Normally two, but recently I have had to use three.

What do you conclude from this story?

- it confirms your suspicion of left heart failure

What would you do now?

- you should find out more about the palpitation

What questions would you ask?

You ask:	*Mrs. Gibson answers:*
Tell me more about this palpitation Mrs. Gibson?	I can feel fluttering and thumping inside my chest.
What do you mean by fluttering?	My heart is beating much too rapidly.
You say you get it when you exert yourself, but isn't it normal for your heart to speed up on exertion?	Yes, I know that doctor, but this is quite different.
In what way is it different?	Well for one thing, it doesn't build up. It just suddenly races off as though someone had pressed a button.
Does it stop that way too?	Sometimes. Other times it just wears off and I really couldn't say exactly when it had stopped.
How fast is it?	It seems to vary. Sometimes it is very rapid and regular. (She indicates about 160 per minute.) Sometimes it's all over the place.
You mean it's irregular?	Yes, very.
What about the thumping?	That is quite different. My heart seems to miss beats and to give very strong beats.
When would you get that?	Anytime. It is often troublesome when I am sitting quietly, reading or watching television.
What do you feel?	Sometimes just an odd thump. Sometimes they come in rapid succession and this can be quite alarming.

(See pages 35–37 for further information about taking a history from a patient with palpitation.)

How do you explain these symptoms?

- she is clearly having many different abnormalities of rhythm
- multiple ectopic beats, paroxysmal tachycardia and paroxysmal atrial fibrillation are all suggested by the history

How would you confirm this diagnosis?

170

- by recording an ECG: remembering that the chance of detecting all the abnormalities on an isolated record is not high. A 24-hour tape will probably be required to do this.

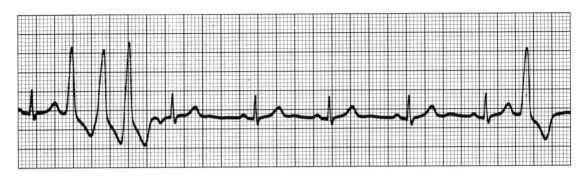

What does the rhythm strip show?

- it shows multiple ventricular ectopic beats, some occurring as a short run

(Ectopic beats: see pages 49, 67 and 73.)

Two excerpts from her 24-hour tape are seen below.

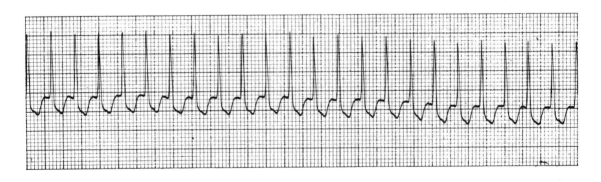

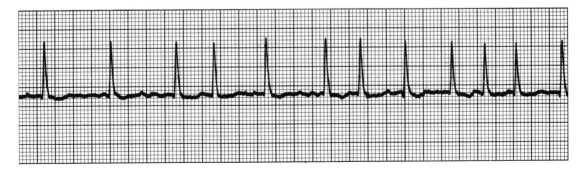

What do they show?

- they confirm your suspicion that she is also having paroxysms of supra-ventricular tachycardia and atrial fibrillation with a rapid ventricular rate

(Supraventricular tachycardia: see page 52. Atrial fibrillation: see page 59.)

What do you think could be causing these disorders of rhythm?

- there is no evidence of clinical coronary heart disease in her past history or current ECG
- her blood pressure in 158/82
- she has no heart murmurs to suggest that she has rheumatic or congenital heart disease
- the only auscultatory abnormality is a loud fourth heart sound that supports your suspicion of heart failure
- an X-ray shows no evidence of a bronchial carcinoma, but reveals that she has considerable cardiomegaly and a little pulmonary congestion

What other possibilities should you keep in mind?

- thyrotoxic heart disease must be excluded. It is often forgotten in the differential diagnosis of such cases, especially when the clinical signs of thyrotoxicosis are not obvious: the so-called masked thyrotoxicosis.

Laboratory tests indicate that this patient does not have hyperthyroidism.

Where do you go from here?

- you are now left with the uncommon forms of heart disease, often grouped together under the title of cardiomyopathies. Unfortunately, this is usually just another way of saying heart disease of unknown aetiology.
- one type that is probably much commoner than many people realise is alcoholic cardiomyopathy, and this turned out to be the diagnosis in Vicki Gibson's case.

SUMMARY

This was a problem about palpitation complicating one of the less common forms of heart disease. It illustrates that symptoms may be caused by a variety of rhythms and that their nature can often be deduced by taking a careful history.

An Old Man with Giddy Turns

John Smith is a 72 year-old widower who lives alone in a council flat. He has always been a very healthy man, but has recently been having giddy turns. They come on without warning, making him feel faint and lightheaded. If he is up and about at the time, he becomes unsteady on his legs and has to sit down till the attack wears off. He has occasionally fallen, but usually has sufficient warning to avoid injuring himself.

The health visitor has asked you to call and see him because he is reluctant to make the long journey to your surgery.

What questions would you ask Mr. Smith when you went to see him?

You ask:	Mr. Smith answers:
Do you ever lose consciousness during an attack?	No.
How long do the attacks last?	Sometimes for just a moment; sometimes for several minutes.
How often do you have them?	I may have several attacks in a row and then none for hours or even days.
Do you ever have warning of an attack?	Yes, sometimes the faint feeling comes on gradually, but more often it is quite sudden.
Has anyone seen one of these turns?	No; I live alone and rarely have visitors nowadays.

What conclusions have you reached so far?

- the history suggests that he may have some disorder of cardiac rate, rhythm or conduction
- vertebrobasilar ischaemia or some type of epilepsy must also be kept in mind

(See page 37 for information about the effects of disordered action of the heart on the efficiency of the cardiovascular system.)

Assuming the former, what further history would you take?

You ask:	Mr. Smith answers:
Do you ever have palpitation, Mr. Smith?	Yes, quite often.
What do you mean by palpitation?	I suddenly feel my heart racing.
How long does it race?	Usually, just for a few minutes and then it suddenly stops again.
How fast is your heart beating when it races?	(He indicates a rate of about 150 per minute.)

(The symptom of palpitation is discussed on pages 35–37.)

What do you conclude from this further information?

- that if he is correct about the rate, his giddy turns are most unlikely to be due to paroxysms of tachycardia

How would you confirm this?

You ask:	Mr. Smith answers:
Do you ever feel giddy when you have palpitation?	No doctor, the two are not related.
Are you ever conscious of your heart beat when you are having an attack of giddiness?	No, never.

Physical examination is unhelpful. His pulse is regular at 68 per minute and his BP is 148/88.

What would you do next?

- you should record an ECG

A rhythm strip is seen below.

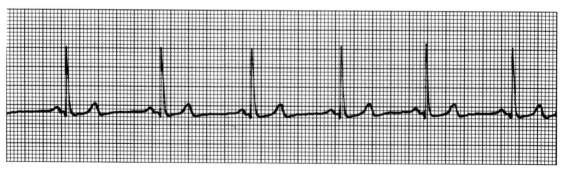

What does it show?

174

- it shows normal sinus rhythm.

Does it help you to decide why he is having giddy turns?

- no

You have an elderly patient whose history indicates that he is having attacks of giddiness and paroxysms of tachycardia. This suggests that his symptoms may be due to a disorder of rate, rhythm or conduction, but the paroxysms do not sound fast enough to be causing giddiness.

Which other disorder might be responsible?

- he may have the sick sinus (bradycardia/tachycardia) syndrome

(The sick sinus syndrome: see page 86.)

What would you do about it?

- you should refer Mr. Smith to the local cardiologist, telling him what you suspect and asking if a 24-hour ECG recording might be helpful in determining the nature of his attacks

The cardiologist agrees that it might and sends you an excerpt from the 24-hour tape for your records.

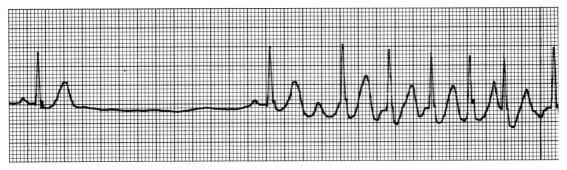

What does it show?

- it confirms your suspicions
- he is having paroxysms of supraventricular tachycardia and also episodes of bradycardia when his heart rate becomes slow enough to be causing symptoms of cerebral ischaemia (some lasted several seconds)

(Supraventricular tachycardia: see page 52. Sinus bradycardia: see page 41.)

How do you think this patient will be treated?

175

- his symptoms will be relieved by the insertion of a permanent pacemaker

(Cardiac pacing: see page 142.)

This may not prevent his palpitations, but these are not really troubling him so far. They can easily be controlled by digoxin or a beta blocker if they do.

SUMMARY

This was a problem about giddy turns occurring in an elderly patient who lived alone. It illustrates that these may be caused by disorders of rate, rhythm or conduction. A careful history and a tape-recorded ECG are often required for the correct diagnosis and treatment.

A Therapeutic Problem

Elizabeth MacSween is a 66 year-old widow who is known to have coronary heart disease. Following a myocardial infarct seven years ago, she was left with a little residual heart failure that was slow to clear. This has been well controlled with digoxin, frusemide and slow-K. She has had no anginal pain since her infarct.

She lives alone in the country and you have received a postal request for a month's supply of her digoxin and frusemide. She enclosed her repeat prescription card as required in your system and you note that she has not been seen for six months.

How often should such patients be seen by their general practitioners?

- elderly patients who are on both digitalis and diuretic therapy should be seen at least every three months for two main reasons: (i) they are at risk of digitalis toxicity; and (ii) they may not need indefinite digitalis therapy or such a powerful diuretic. Research has shown that many elderly patients are taking digoxin unnecessarily.

A copy of this patient's current repeat prescription card is shown below.

	DATE	DRUGS
Name: Elizabeth MacSween	2/1/84	1, 2, 4
The Rowans	30/1/84	2, 3, 4
St. Fergus	28/2/84	1, 2, 4
	28/3/84	2, 4
	26/4/84	1, 2, 3, 4

DRUGS FOR REPEAT PRESCRIPTION

1 Digoxin 0.25mg daily	28
2 Frusemide 40mg daily	28
3 Slow K 600mg t.i.d.	100
4 Mogadon 5mg nocte	28

Having studied the card, what comments have you to make about it?

- the card indicates that she has not been taking her digoxin or her potassium supplement regularly

You ask your receptionist to send Mrs. MacSween an appointment to see you soon. She comes to your surgery a few days later.

What aspects of the case would you want to explore with Mrs. MacSween?

- you would want to find out if she still has any symptoms suggesting heart failure

You ask:	Mrs. MacSween answers:
Do you have breathlessness or a cough on exertion or in bed at night?	I am very well, doctor, and have no trouble with my breathing now.
How many pillows do you sleep with?	One.
Do your ankles ever swell?	No.

- you would want to find out about symptoms of digitalis toxicity or potassium deficiency

You ask:	Mrs. MacSween answers:
Do you enjoy your food?	I have a good appetite so long as I don't take too many of these large yellow pills.
Do you ever feel sick?	The pills often give me a pain in my stomach, but I never feel sick.
Have you had any diarrhoea?	I don't have any trouble with my bowels.
Any undue fatigue and malaise or headaches?	No.

What conclusions do you draw from the history?

- she appears to be keeping well and has no symptoms of heart failure
- as she seems none the worse for missing out the digoxin and potassium supplement, you should question the necessity for continuing this therapy

(Digoxin therapy: see pages 132.)

How would you determine whether or not it is still necessary?

You ask:	Mrs. MacSween answers:
How do you feel when you are not taking your digoxin tablets?	I feel fine, but after a week or so my heart races a bit.
What do you mean 'your heart races a bit'?	It just appears to be going faster.
Is it fast all the time?	Yes, but especially when I am hurrying.

Further questioning is not rewarding so you examine her and find no abnormality. The following ECG is recorded.

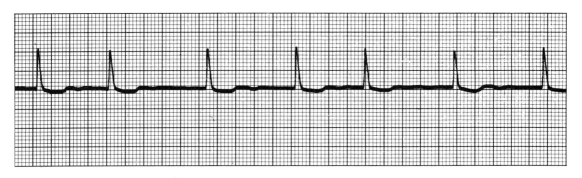

What rhythm does it reveal?

- it reveals that she has atrial fibrillation with a slow, almost regular, ventricular response that could easily be mistaken for sinus rhythm at the bedside

(Atrial fibrillation: see page 59.)

Does this finding help to explain her symptoms?

- yes, it does

When she stops taking digoxin her AV block slowly lessens, more supra-ventricular impulses are conducted to the ventricles and her heart rate increases.

How does this knowledge influence your management of Mrs. MacSween's case?

- without an ECG, it would have been tempting to stop all her tablets and see how she got on without them
- the ECG reveals that she has atrial fibrillation, and although she no longer requires digoxin to control heart failure, her history suggests that she requires it to control her ventricular rate
- you should tell her that you are going to stop the diuretic and slow K for a trial period and explain why she must keep taking the digoxin tablets

SUMMARY

This was a problem about the management of an elderly woman on long-term maintenance therapy for heart failure. It illustrates the need to keep such patients under constant review to make certain that their treatment is still necessary.

HOSPITAL DOCTOR PROBLEMS

A Woman Who Collapsed in the Street

You are asked to see a 75 year-old woman in the Admission Department. She had collapsed in the street and had been brought to hospital by ambulance in response to a 999 call.

The patient is now fully conscious and remembers very little about the episode. She feels well and has no complaints.

Physical examination reveals little of note except for a rather slow pulse of about 40 per minute, a cut above the left eyebrow and bruising over the left shoulder and hip. Her past history tells of frequent giddy attacks during the last year and several blackouts during the last few months.

She has been seen at the medical out-patient department where urine analysis and blood sugars were found to be normal, and at the neurological clinic where a brain scan and EEG revealed no abnormality.

What further history do you wish to have and why?

You ask:	*The patient answers:*
Do you actually lose consciousness during a blackout?	Yes.
Is the loss of consciousness sudden?	Yes.
Did you injure yourself when you fell to the ground?	Yes.

This information is important because many people who are said to have 'blackouts' do not actually lose consciousness. Even when they do, they often have enough warning to sit down or lie down before they lose consciousness. Genuine 'drop attacks', where patients are fully conscious one moment and flat on their face the next, usually cause injury when the patient falls (bruises, cuts, burns etc.).

How long do the attacks last?	Fifteen to twenty seconds.

This information is important in differential diagnosis. Brain damage and death occur 3 to 4 minutes after sudden cessation of cardiac output. So, if the attacks are prolonged, they cannot be due to Adams-Stokes seizures which are always short-lived, self-terminating and usually last for less than 30 seconds.

Has anyone witnessed an attack and the recovery phase that follows it?	My sister says that I just suddenly fall to the ground without warning and then wake up again a few moments later.

180

Information from an eye witness is always helpful because it confirms or refutes that the loss of consciousness was sudden and unexpected, and that recovery was rapid and spontaneous. This is important in the differential diagnosis of such things as vasovagal attacks, giddiness with confusion, epileptic seizures, etc.

During an Adams-Stokes attack, the patient may be pale or cyanosed and is always pulseless. Recovery is rapid and spontaneous with return of consciousness and the heart beat. Sometimes flushing is seen as the blood begins to flow again through the dilated peripheral capillary network. Convulsions may occur in prolonged attacks or when attacks recur frequently.

(See pages 33–38 for more about the effects of disordered action of the heart on the cardiovascular system.)

From the information you have been given, what do you think is the probable diagnosis in this case?

• complete heart block

If an elderly person has a 'drop attack' and is injured when falling to the ground, an Adams-Stokes attack should be assumed until proved otherwise.

Her ECG is shown below.

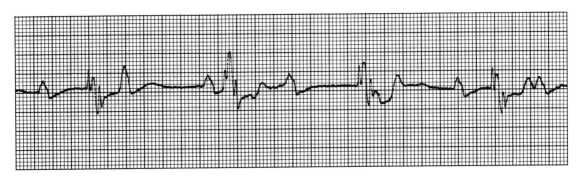

Does this ECG confirm your diagnosis?

• yes it does; it shows complete heart block

Remember that in patients who have unstable block, the resting record does not always show complete block. Adams-Stokes attacks often occur when the rhythm changes into and out of complete block.

(Complete heart block: see page 99.)

If this patient's history had suggested giddy turns rather than 'drop attacks', what disorders of rate, rhythm or conduction might have been responsible?

- any paroxysmal tachycardia with a very rapid ventricular rate
- the sick sinus (tachycardia/bradycardia) syndrome
- extreme sinus bradycardia, possibly with coupled rhythm when each normal beat is followed by an ectopic beat that produces no significant cardiac output and is not transmitted to the pulse
- sinus arrest

(Paroxysmal tachycardias: see pages 52, 68 and 177. The sick sinus syndrome: see page 86. Sinus bradycardia: see page 41. Sinus arrest: see page 84.)

Here are the ECGs of two elderly patients with giddy turns:

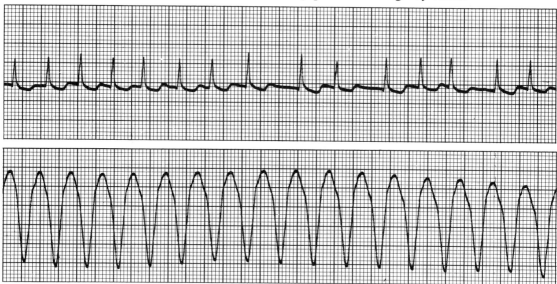

What do they show?

- atrial fibrillation
- ventricular tachycardia

(Atrial fibrillation: see page 59. Ventricular tachycardia: see page 77.)

How would you treat this patient in whom you have diagnosed complete heart block?

- admit her to hospital to prevent serious injury from sudden loss of consciousness
- monitor her ECG and carry out 24-hour tape recordings to see whether or not the block is stable and to study the heart rate at rest and on exercise
- arrange to insert a permanent pacemaker

(The treatment of complete heart block: see page 101. Cardiac pacing: see page 142.)

Is any form of non-invasive medical treatment likely to be an effective alternative to the insertion of a pacemaker?

- not really

Isoprenaline (Saventrine) sometimes relieves the symptoms of low cardiac output by increasing the ventricular rate, but it is not always effective and may cause dangerous ventricular dysrhythmias.

Occasionally, as noted above, when the block is unstable, Adams-Stokes attacks occur when the rhythm changes into and out of complete heart block. In these circumstances, digoxin, by increasing the delay in conduction through the AV junctional tissues, may relieve symptoms by making the block permanent.

(Isoprenaline therapy: see page 136. Digoxin therapy: see page 132.)

Is it cost-effective to implant an expensive pacemaker in a person of this age?

- yes, it is, even for a relatively short time

Patients with complete heart block are mostly elderly and have outlived most of the other common health hazards. Many of them live alone. Once symptoms develop, they become dependent upon others and are afraid to move about on their own. This often necessitates many years of expensive hospital or institutional care. With a pacemaker they soon regain confidence and can return to a normal or near-normal life in the community.

What continuing care is required after the pacemaker is inserted?

- she must attend a pacemaker clinic every six months to have her pacemaker checked. Nowadays with lithium batteries, they should last for at least ten years.
- no special precautions with electrical appliances, etc. are necessary with current models
- patients with pacemakers should be encouraged to lead normal lives, and may even continue to drive a motor car if certified fit to do so by a cardiologist
- when they die, the pacemaker clinic should be notified immediately so that the pacemaker can be removed before burial or cremation

(The supervision and follow-up of patients after a pacemaker has been inserted is detailed on page 144.)

SUMMARY

This was a problem about blackouts in an elderly patient who had been falling and injuring herself when she lost consciousness. It illustrates that complete heart block with Adams-Stokes attacks are a likely cause of such symptoms and that the insertion of a cardiac pacemaker is the cost-effective treatment of choice.

Death in the Night

You are called to the ward in the middle of the night to see a 53 year-old man who had been transferred from the coronary care unit the previous day. He had cried out for a nurse, but, by the time she arrived, had slumped forward in bed and appeared to be dead. She immediately summoned help.

When you get there, just ahead of the cardiac arrest trolley, closed-chest cardiac massage with mouth-to-mouth breathing is already in progress.

What are the likely causes of this patient's collapse?

- ventricular fibrillation (VF)
- asystolic arrest
- very rapid ventricular tachycardia (VT)
- pulmonary embolism

(Ventricular fibrillation: see page 80. Asystolic arrest: see page 82. Ventricular tachycardia: see page 77.)

On arrival, would you: record an ECG to determine the nature of the abnormal rhythm or commence cardiac resuscitation immediately?

- you should commence treatment immediately

In this situation, seconds are precious. The patient is at risk of further brain damage and death. You should assume that the patient has ventricular fibrillation without waiting for an ECG to confirm the diagnosis, unless the defibrillator happens to have a built-in facility to display the ECG when the electrodes are applied to the chest wall.

What action should you take?

- stop the resuscitation temporarily
- confirm the absence of a pulse or heart beat
- thump the lower sternum forcefully once or twice with a clenched fist
- give a DC shock *immediately* if the heart beat does not return

(Cardioversion: see page 130.)

What subsidiary instructions should be given simultaneously?

184

- establish a satisfactory airway and supply oxygen after the shock has been given
- set up an IV line
- prepare to infuse 8.4% sodium bicarbonate (1ml/kg)
- make ready two syringes – one containing 10ml 1:10,000 adrenaline, the other 10ml 10% calcium chloride
- attach electrodes so that an ECG can be recorded immediately after the shock

Remember to make sure that no-one is touching the patient or the bed when the shock is given.

(The treatment of cardiac arrest: see page 128.)

What would be the likely outcome of a DC shock if the patient has: (a) ventricular fibrillation, (b) asystolic arrest, (c) very rapid ventricular tachycardia?

(a) restoration of normal rhythm (conversion to asystolic arrest becomes more likely in the later stages of the illness),
(b) no change,
(c) restoration of normal rhythm.

(See pages 81, 82 and 79 for the treatment of these three conditions.)

Following a DC shock, normal rhythm is restored in this patient.

What would you do next?

- give a bolus of 100mg lignocaine IV over two minutes
- follow this with a lignocaine infusion of 2mg per minute
- connect the patient to a monitor so that his ECG can be observed continuously
- arrange for him to return to coronary care

(Lignocaine therapy: see page 138.)

Soon after treatment has commenced the patient again slumps forward unconscious. This time the rhythm, seen below, appears on the oscilloscope.

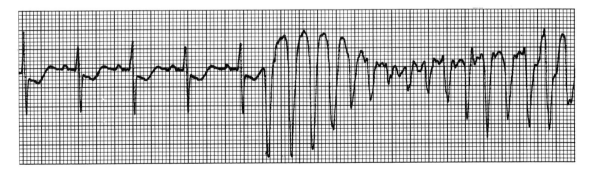

What does it show?

- it shows ventricular fibrillation

What would you do now?

- you should repeat the DC shock

and if normal rhythm is restored:

- give another 100mg bolus of lignocaine IV
- increase the concentration of lignocaine in the infusion to 3mg per minute

If the patient has further VF or VT despite increasing doses of lignocaine, what would you do next?

- several other drugs can be used instead of lignocaine. At present, either mexiletine or disopyramide would be the first choice.

(Mexiletine therapy: see page 140. Disopyramide therapy: see page 134.)

Both are equally effective in suppressing ventricular dysrhythmias, but have unpleasant side effects when compared with lignocaine, which for this reason, is still the drug of first choice.

If the ECG below had appeared following the DC shock, what diagnosis would you have made? And what would you do in these circumstances?

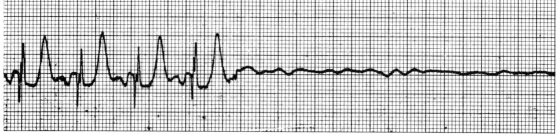

- you would conclude that the shock had converted the ventricular fibrillation into asystolic arrest
- you should: (i) inject 10ml 1:10,000 adrenaline and 10ml 10% calcium chloride IV directly into the heart and (ii) insert a temporary pacemaker

Remember, however, that the treatment of asystolic arrest is only occasionally successful.

SUMMARY

This was a problem about cardiac arrest in a patient who had had a fairly recent myocardial infarct. It illustrates that ventricular fibrillation should be assumed in these circumstances. Cardiac resuscitation should be started immediately and a DC shock given without delay.

186

An Elderly Patient with Heart Failure

A female patient aged 62 years, who has only recently come to live in the district, is admitted to your ward for investigation and treatment. She is known to have long-standing rheumatic heart disease (mitral incompetence and stenosis). Although her symptoms have not warranted valve replacement, she has been on medical treatment with digoxin and bendrofluazide for many years. Previous ECGs are not available.

Recently, during an acute respiratory illness, her GP prescribed an antibiotic. This cleared up the secondary infection, but caused severe diarrhoea. Following this, she developed persistent crepitations at both lung bases, a little hepatomegaly and slight ankle oedema.

You have been asked to work up her case.

What thoughts should be running through your mind at this stage?

- that chest infection frequently causes heart failure in patients with chronic rheumatic heart disease
- that diarrhoea may have upset her fluid and electrolyte balance

Because of the heart failure, her diuretic was changed to frusemide 40mg b.d. but, despite a good diuresis, she seemed worse rather than better.

Her heart rate was rapid and irregular and at around 120 per minute. So, thinking she had atrial fibrillation, the doctor increased her daily dose of digoxin from 0.25mg to 0.50mg for a few days. As a result, her heart rate became regular and fell to 70 per minute. Despite this, her condition continued to deteriorate and she was sent to the local cottage hospital.

On admission, she was orthopnoeic and her signs of heart failure persisted. An ECG showed rapid regular P waves, every second one of which was followed by a QRS complex. A diagnosis of atrial flutter was made and quinidine prescribed without benefit.

She has now been transferred to a nearby teaching hospital where the following ECG was recorded.

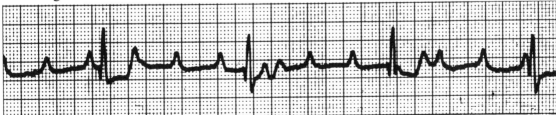

What abnormality does it show?

187

- atrial tachycardia with complete AV block

The spikey P waves recur regularly at a rate of 125 per minute. The broad QRS complexes recur regularly at a rate of 40 per minute. The P waves and the QRS complexes bear no relationship to each other.

(Atrial tachycardia with AV block: see page 56.)

What rhythm do you think the GP had suspected when he found a rapid irregular pulse and increased her dose of digoxin?

- atrial fibrillation with a rapid ventricular rate

(Atrial fibrillation: see page 59.)

What simple bedside tests might have suggested that he was wrong?

- a pulse deficit is nearly always present in atrial fibrillation when the ventricular rate is rapid. In this patient, the heart and pulse rates would have been the same.
    When a disorder of rate, rhythm or conduction is suspected, always count both the heart rate and the pulse rate carefully over at least 30 seconds and preferably for a full minute (see page 37).
- vagal stimulation (carotid sinus massage) might have caused slowing of the ventricular rate

(Vagal stimulation: see page 154.)

What abnormality of rhythm do you think had been present when the GP diagnosed atrial fibrillation?

- atrial tachycardia with a varying degree of AV block

What was the likely cause of this abnormality?

- initially, loss of fluid and potassium resulting from the diarrhoea
- later, this was aggravated by changing to a more powerful diuretic
- finally, by increasing rather than decreasing the dose of digoxin

Why did the ventricular rate fall after extra digoxin?

- because the extra digoxin increased the degree of block in the AV junctional tissues and fewer of the supraventricular impulses were conducted to the ventricles

Why did the patient's condition deteriorate despite the fall in heart rate?

- because she was already suffering from the toxic effects of digitalis: even on the smaller dose

What features on the first ECG should have indicated that she did not have atrial flutter?

- the relatively slow atrial rate of 125 per minute. In atrial flutter, the atrial rate varies between 280 and 320 per minute
- the flat iso-electric baseline between the regularly recurring P waves. In atrial flutter it usually has the characteristic saw-toothed appearance seen below.

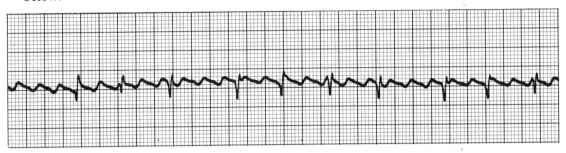

(Atrial flutter: see page 62.)

The referral letter that came with the patient had suggested that she might require cardioversion.

Would you consider cardioversion as a possible method of treatment for atrial tachycardia in this case?

- certainly not

Cardioversion should never be used in patients suffering from digitalis toxicity. In such circumstances, a DC shock may provoke dangerous ventricular dysrhythmias.

(Cardioversion: see page 130.)

What treatment would you advise?

- stop the digoxin
- give a potassium supplement
- in this case, use IV phenytoin as serious haemodynamic deterioration has already taken place. Oral phenytoin acts too slowly.
- sometimes, stopping the digoxin may be all that is required

(Phenytoin therapy: see page 145.)

SUMMARY

This was a problem about heart failure that got worse instead of better despite what appeared to be adequate medical treatment. It illustrates that abnormalities of rhythm may be caused by too much digoxin, and that they are often difficult or impossible to diagnose at the bedside without the help of an ECG. Digitalis toxicity is especially likely to occur in older patients following an upset in their fluid and electrolyte balance.

An Emergency in the Theatre Suite

You are called to the gynaecological operating theatre to see a 56 year-old woman who is said to have had a cardiac arrest during induction of anaesthesia for diagnostic curettage to determine the cause of postmenopausal bleeding.

She had made a good recovery from an anterior myocardial infarction three and a half months ago and appeared to be well when examined in the ward on the previous day.

What should you be thinking as you make your way to the theatre suite?

- that ventricular fibrillation is a common cause of cardiac arrest during surgery, especially in patients with coronary heart disease who have had a fairly recent myocardial infarction

When you arrive in theatre, cardiac massage is in progress. A peripheral pulse is palpable each time her chest is compressed and she is being adequately ventilated with 100% oxygen. Sodium bicarbonate 25ml 8%; 250mg aminophyline; 200mg hydrocortisone and 2.5mg neostigmine have been given.

Although there are facilities for monitoring the ECG in the anaesthetic room, nothing is visible on the oscilloscope.

You are told that she was anaesthetised with 500mg thiopentone, 50mg suxamethomium and 80mg gallamine. During intubation, many supra-ventricular and ventricular ectopic beats were observed. She developed bronchospasm and became cyanosed. The endotracheal tube was withdrawn and when re-inserted, the QRS complexes became progressively slower and then appeared to stop. It is possible that one of the ECG electrodes became loosened while preparations were being made for emergency action.

The likelihood of cardiac arrest was strengthened by the fact that no peripheral pulses could be felt and her blood pressure became unrecordable.

(Cardiac arrest and its treatment: see page 128.)

Would you assume that she had ventricular fibrillation (VF) and give an immediate DC shock?

- no

Although VF is a common cause of cardiac arrest during surgery, especially in patients with coronary heart disease who have fairly recent myocardial infarction, she has had effective resuscitation throughout. Also, you know that disturbances of rate, rhythm and conduction are common during the induction of anaesthesia. So, under these circumstances, it would be reasonable to study an ECG before taking further action.

The following appeared on the oscilloscope when the leads were reconnected.

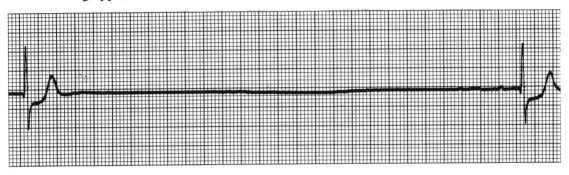

What does it show?

- it shows extreme bradycardia

(Sinus bradycardia: see page 41.)

How do you explain this and what has been the likely sequence of events?

- the introduction of an endotracheal tube acted as a powerful vagal stimulant. The tube was withdrawn and then re-inserted. This had almost certainly caused profound slowing of the heart and probably a period of asystole.

How would you have treated such a case?

- the measures described in the history are the correct treatment
- the condition is usually brief and self-terminating
- when it lasts a longer time, as in this case, cardiac resuscitation should be commenced to maintain the circulation during the temporary cessation of cardiac output
- it is always worthwhile striking the lower sternum once or twice with a clenched fist before starting the cardiac massage

(The treatment of sinus bradycardia: see page 43.)

What would you do now?

- give IV atropine 0.6mg to speed up the heart rate and repeat this after ten minutes if spontaneous recovery is delayed

(Atropine therapy: see page 124.)

Soon after the atropine had been given, the following ECG was recorded.

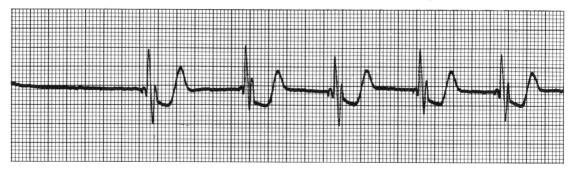

What would you conclude from this record?

- that the treatment had been successful
- though clearly not sinus rhythm, the heart rate is now back to normal

What would you have done if the first ECG had shown no QRS complexes?

- given another dose of sodium bicarbonate and 0.6mg of atropine intravenously.
- continued with cardiac massage and ventilation

If QRS complexes did not appear soon, what would you have done next?

- injected 5ml, 1:10,000 adrenaline and 10ml, 10% calcium chloride intravenously or, if you were unhappy about the cardiac output being achieved by cardiac massage, directly into the heart
- inserted a cardiac pacemaker, if one was available

With this type of cardiac arrest, however, it is unlikely that such measures would be necessary. The condition is usually self-terminating in the absence of further vagal stimulation.

(Ventricular standstill: see page 82.)

SUMMARY

This was a problem about cardiac arrest occurring during the induction of anaesthesia. It illustrates that intense vagal stimulation may cause profound bradycardia or even asystole. Although alarming, the disturbance is usually transitory and, provided the circulation is maintained when necessary, does not call for the heroic measures normally required in cases of cardiac arrest.

The treatment of cardiac emergencies in theatre is often complicated by the combined effect of several powerful anaesthetic agents, each of which may affect the cardiovascular system in a variety of ways. It did not cause concern in this patient, but must always be kept in mind when ordering therapy in such circumstances.

A Schoolgirl with Tachycardia

You are called to the Admission Department to see a 16 year-old girl who has been brought from school complaining of palpitation, associated with dizziness, nausea and blurred vision.

On examination, she looks pale and distressed. Her heart rate is too rapid to count accurately, but is certainly more than 180 per minute. Her blood pressure is 80/50.

(This symptom, palpitation, is discussed on pages 35–37.)

What further history would you wish to have about the nature of the attack?

You ask:	*The girl answers:*
How long have you had it?	It started about two hours ago.
What were you doing at the time?	I was sitting quietly in the classroom.
How did it start?	Suddenly. One moment I felt fine. The next, I felt my heart racing in my chest and a pounding in my head and neck.
Have you ever had anything like this before?	Yes. I have been having similar attacks, about ten a year since I was 7 years old.
How long do they last?	Always for several hours, sometimes nearly all day.
How do they stop?	Although they always start suddenly they wear off gradually if I lie down quietly in a darkened room. I really couldn't say exactly when an attack stops.

From this history, what do you think is the probable cause of her symptoms?

- in the absence of severe organic heart disease, it is almost certain to be supraventricular tachycardia

How would you try to exclude serious heart disease?

- you should not try to do so at this stage

Her heart rate is much too fast and, as a result, her circulation is much too compromised to draw any meaningful conclusions from a detailed examination of her cardiovascular system.

What should you do at this stage?

193

- you should establish the nature of the paroxysm by recording an ECG and, having done so, you should decide how to stop it

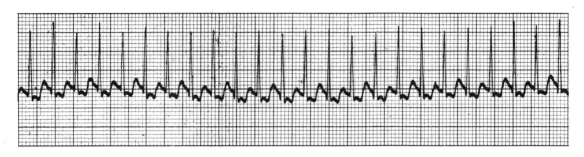

What diagnosis would you make from this ECG?

- supraventricular tachycardia: rate 240 per minute

(Supraventricular tachycardia: see page 52.)

Before deciding about treatment what further questions would you ask?

You ask:	*The girl answers:*
What treatment have you had since the attacks started nine years ago?	Soon after the attacks started, my doctor prescribed digoxin tablets, but they didn't seem to do much good, so I stopped taking them.
	A few months ago, Dad took me back to the doctor after I had an attack that lasted all the day before. The doctor prescribed sotalol 80mg twice daily, but I stopped taking it after two weeks.
Are you having any treatment at present?	I am having no treatment at present?

Would you take active steps to terminate this attack?

- yes, you should try to stop it

Why should you, when you know from the history that it will eventually stop spontaneously?

Because:
- the heart rate is very rapid
- the attacks usually last a long time
- she already has symptoms of inadequate cardiac output

How would you stop the tachycardia?

194

- if vagal stimulation is ineffective and she is having no other drugs, you should give 5mg IV verapamil (Cordilox) under ECG control and repeat this dose once or twice if necessary

(Verapamil therapy: see page 156.)

In this case, the first dose terminated the attack and the following ECG was recorded.

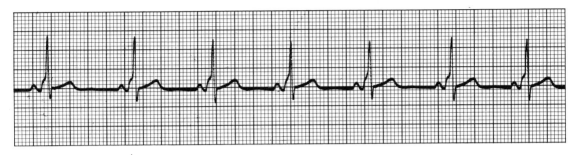

What does it show?

- a short PR interval (0.08 seconds) and a broad QRS complex caused by an early delta wave. She has pre-excitation.

(Ventricular pre-excitation: see page 106.)

A careful physical examination carried out the next day revealed no abnormality in her cardiovascular system. A diagnosis of Wolff-Parkinson-White syndrome with re-entrant tachycardia is appropriate and the question of prophylactic treatment arises.

Do you think it necessary to prescribe daily treatment when, on average, she has less than one attack per month?

- in many cases. the answer would be no

Decisions about prophylactic treatment, however, depend not only upon the frequency of attacks, but also upon their duration and severity.

In this case, the heart rate is 240 per minute during paroxysms and they often last for many hours. As evidenced by her symptoms, even a healthy heart cannot maintain an adequate circulation for long under these circumstances, so suppressive therapy is necessary.

When prescribing, remember that very rapid tachycardia in patients with the WPW syndrome is sometimes difficult to control and that the first drug tried may not be effective.

(Therapeutic principles are discussed on page 119.)

What treatment would you advise for this girl?

195

- the beta blocker sotalol (Beta-Cardone; Sotacor) was not given a fair trial and it, or some similar preparation, should be used again as the drug of first choice, starting with 80mg b.d. and increasing, if necessary, to a maximum of 240 mg per day.
- if this is not successful, verapamil (Cordilox) could be tried. Although less effective when given orally than when used intravenously, it is beneficial in some cases. Start with 40mg t.d.s. and increase as necessary to two or three times this dose.
- amiodarone (Cordarone X) may prevent paroxysms when other drugs have failed. It differs from most others in that you start with the maximum dose, 200mg t.d.s. for at least one week and then gradually reduce the dose to 200mg per day.

(Beta blocker therapy: see page 125. Verapamil therapy: see page 156. Amiodarone therapy: see page 122.)

SUMMARY

This was a problem about paroxysmal supraventricular tachycardia in an apparently healthy girl. It illustrates that decisions about the nature of the abnormality, and whether or not it requires treatment, can be made by taking a careful history.

A Man Conscious of his Heart Beat

You have been asked to see a lean 54 year-old man in the out-patient department. During the last two years he has become a little breathless on exertion, has lost some weight and has often been conscious of the fact that his heart beats rapidly and forcefully in response to effort or emotion. For six months he has been increasingly troubled by palpitation, which he describes as a rapid and irregular fluttering sensation behind his breastbone. At first, it occurred infrequently and lasted for only a few minutes. Recently, it has troubled him nearly every day and has often lasted for several hours.

His general practitioner noted that he had an irregular pulse of 120 per minute. He could find no obvious cause for the abnormal rhythm, but prescribed digoxin in 0.25mg b.d. to control the rapid rate. Two weeks later the patient was no better and the ventricular rate was no slower, so he referred the patient to hospital for advice and treatment.

After examining him carefully, like the GP, you can find no obvious cause for his symptoms.

His skin is warm. He has a rapid regular pulse of 125 per minute. His blood pressure is 158/68. His heart is slightly enlarged and his first heart sound is loud and slapping.

His ECG is shown below.

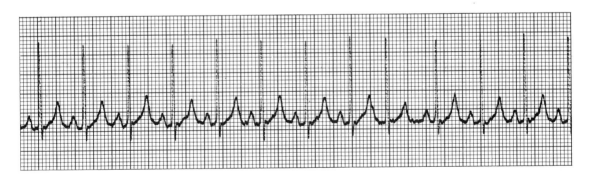

What does it show?

• it shows sinus tachycardia

(Sinus tachycardia: see page 44.)

Fortunately, the ECG seen overleaf, which was recorded by the GP, was enclosed with the referral letter.

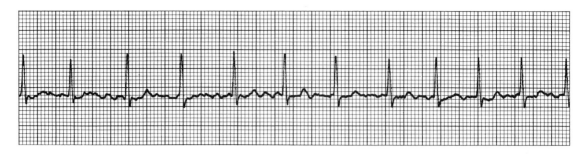

From the patient's history and these two ECG's, what diagnosis can you make?

- that he is suffering from paroxysmal atrial fibrillation

(Atrial fibrillation: see page 59.)

What are the most common causes of this disorder in a man of his age?

- coronary heart disease
- hypertensive heart disease
- rheumatic heart disease

As there is no evidence of any of these conditions in this case, what other diagnosis should you consider?

- thyrotoxic heart disease

Does the absence of exophthalmos, lid lag, tremor, enlargement of the thyroid gland or other obvious signs of thyrotoxicosis exclude such a diagnosis?

- no

So-called 'masked thyrotoxicosis' may well be present and is commonly overlooked.

Which of his clinical features support the possibility of thyrotoxicosis?

- his age
- loss of weight without anorexia
- the warm skin
- sinus tachycardia
- an overactive, slightly enlarged heart
- a high pulse pressure
- paroxysmal atrial fibrillation with a rapid ventricular rate that did not respond to digoxin

What other disorders of rhythm may cause irregular palpitation?

198

None is common, but these two possibilities should be kept in mind:
- multiple ectopic beats
- atrial flutter with a frequently changing degree of AV block

(Ectopic beats: see pages 49, 67, and 73. Atrial flutter: see page 62.)

Laboratory tests confirm that this patient is thyrotoxic. How would you treat his abnormal rhythm?

- you should not treat the abnormal rhythm. You should treat its cause, the thyrotoxicosis.

In a case like this, the paroxysmal atrial fibrillation and the sinus tachycardia will cease to be a problem once the thyrotoxicosis is under control.

If he had had atrial fibrillation as an established rhythm, and signs of heart failure, what would you have done?

- used digoxin and diuretics to treat the heart failure, and

- given a beta blocker to help control the ventricular rate until the antithyroid therapy took effect

(Digoxin therapy: see page 132. Beta blocker therapy: see page 125.)

If the atrial fibrillation had persisted after he became euthyroid, what would you have done?

- restored sinus rhythm with a DC shock

(Cardioversion: see page 130.)

SUMMARY

This was a problem about palpitation in a middle-aged patient that occurred without obvious cause and failed to respond to conventional therapy. It illustrates that thyrotoxicosis should always be kept in mind as a possible cause of such symptoms, even when it is not clinically obvious.

Treatment, at least in the first instance, should be concentrated not upon the abnormal rhythm, but upon its cause.

NURSE PROBLEMS

A Problem in Coronary Care

While on duty in the coronary care unit, you notice that a patient who was admitted the previous day with a recent inferior myocardial infarct develops the following ECG.

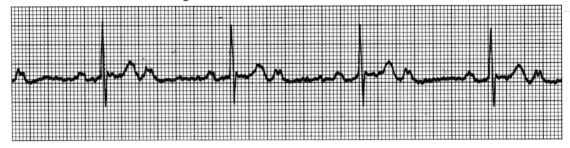

What abnormality does it show?

- it shows 2:1 heart block

What are the atrial and ventricular rates?

- the atrial rate is 96 per minute
- the ventricular rate is 48 per minute

(Methods of counting the heart rate from an ECG are described on pages 10–12.)

Where does 2:1 heart block fit into the classification of conduction defects?

- it is second degree atrioventricular block, Type II

What other kind of AV block is included under this heading?

- the one seen below, where ventricular complexes fail to appear at random and without warning

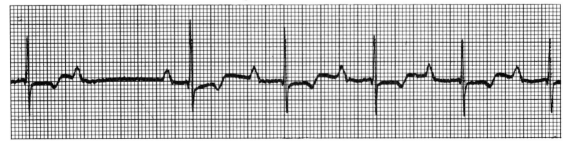

(Second degree heart block, Type II: see page 93.)

You report by telephone to the doctor that the patient has developed 2:1 block. What questions would you expect him to ask?

- What is the ventricular rate?
- Has the patient's clinical condition deteriorated?
- Have the QRS complexes broadened?

You say that the rate is 43 per minute and that there has been no change in the patient's clinical condition or in the QRS complexes.

Why does he then ask you merely to observe carefully and report further developments?

- because conduction defects are not uncommon after inferior infarction
- they are usually transient and often relatively benign

What would you have expected him to say if the patient had had a recent anterior infarct?

- make immediate preparations for the insertion of a temporary pacing catheter

Why is there such a difference between the way in which these situations are managed?

- high grade heart block in recent anterior infarction is a sign of extensive myocardial damage and may harbinger the sudden onset of extreme bradycardia or asystole
- in these circumstances, the presence of a pacemaker 'in situ' may be life-saving

A little later the ECG changes again.

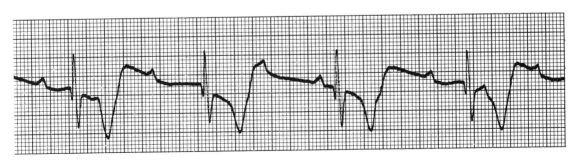

(The treatment of second degree block complicating acute myocardial infarction is discussed on page 95.)

What has happened this time?

201

● the patient has developed third degree (complete) heart block

(Third degree block: see page 99)

How would you expect the doctor to react to this information?

● in much the same way that he reacted before

In inferior infarction, the abnormality itself does not require treatment, only its haemodynamic consequences. So, if the patient appears well and the cardiac output remains adequate, no specific treatment is required.

Should the patient's condition deteriorate, temporary cardiac pacing would be carried out without delay.

(The treatment of third degree block complicating acute myocardial infarction is discussed on page 101.)

SUMMARY

This was a problem about the progressive development of heart block following inferior myocardial infarction.

It illustrates that in inferior infarcts, treatment is unnecessary unless the abnormality of conduction causes deterioration in the patient's clinical condition.

An Intensive Care Emergency

You are on duty in the intensive care unit with a 46 year-old patient who had a large atrial septal defect closed six hours ago. This is a copy of her ECG.

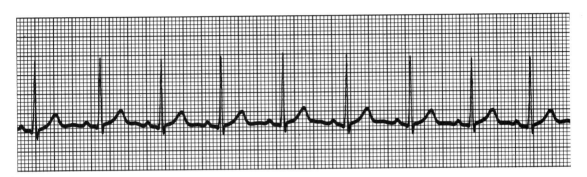

What does it show?

• it shows normal sinus rhythm

(Normal sinus rhythm: see page 39.)

What is the ventricular rate?

• the ventricular rate is 92 per minute

(Methods of calculating the heart rate are described on pages 10–12.)

While you are watching the oscilloscope, the tracing changes to the one seen below.

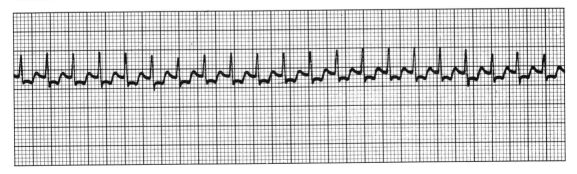

What has happened?

- she has developed supraventricular tachycardia

(Supraventricular tachycardia: see page 52.)

What is the ventricular rate now?

- it has increased to 210 per minute

Would you report this change to the surgical staff, or would you wait to tell them about it when they pay a visit that is due within the hour?

- you should report it at once

Why would it be wrong to wait?

- because a ventricular rate of 210 in a patient of this age who has just had open heart surgery may cause acute heart failure

(The effect of disordered action of the heart on the cardiovascular system is discussed on pages 37–38.)

How would you expect your patient to be treated?

- this would depend upon her clinical condition. If it had not deteriorated and she had not already had digitalis, she could be given intravenous digoxin or intravenous verapamil.
- alternatively, she could be given one of the beta blockers that can be used intravenously

(Digoxin, page 132; verapamil, page 156; beta blockers: page 125.)

Why is it important to find out if a patient is taking digitalis or beta blockers before giving IV verapamil?

- because verapamil has a powerful inotropic effect when given with a beta blocker and may cause asystole when given to digitalised patients

If her condition had already deteriorated by the time the doctors arrived or if they were afraid that it might do so, what would you expect them to do?

- they would restore sinus rhythm as rapidly as possible by giving a DC shock. A DC shock was the treatment used in this case.

(Cardioversion: see page 130.)

Following the shock, her ECG changed again.

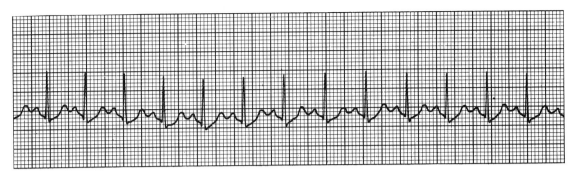

What does it show now?

- the paroxysm has been terminated
- she now has sinus tachycardia

(Sinus tachycardia: see page 44.)

What continuing therapy might be used to prevent further paroxysms of tachycardia?

- digoxin or a beta blocking drug should be given orally, possibly with an initial IV loading dose
- should these prove ineffective, quinidine, disopyramide or amiodarone could be tried

(Digoxin, page 132; beta blockers, page 125; quinidine, page 150; disopyramide, page 134; amiodarone, page 122.)

What simple therapeutic measure has been forgotten in this case?

- no one has suggested that the paroxysm might be terminated by vagal stimulation

How might this be carried out?

- by carotid sinus massage
- by gagging
- by performing Valsalva's manoeuvre

(Vagal stimulation: see page 154.)

SUMMARY

This was a problem about a paroxysm of supraventricular tachycardia occurring in a patient who had just had open heart surgery. It illustrates the importance of considering not only the nature of the disorder, but also the state of the heart itself. In these circumstances, a very rapid rate was a serious complication that might have caused acute heart failure, so no time was lost in restoring normal rhythm.

A Recent Myocardial Infarct

You are on duty in the emergency admission area and a patient with a recent myocardial infarct is having his ECG monitored. You notice that an occasional abnormality of rhythm is becoming increasingly frequent and record a strip for analysis.

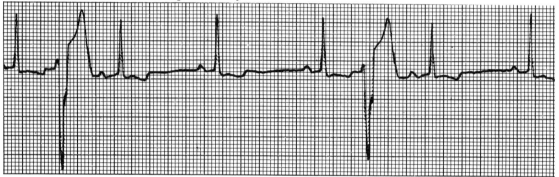

What is the abnormality?

- the patient is having frequent ventricular ectopic beats

(Ventricular ectopic beats: see page 73.)

Should you report these?

- no

Such ventricular ectopic beats are common following myocardial infarction and do not require treatment.

Later you notice a change in the pattern of the ectopic beats.

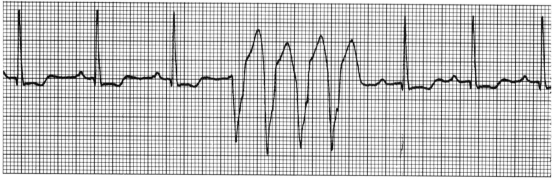

206

What is happening now?

- the patient is having short runs of consecutive ventricular ectopic beats or short paroxysms of ventricular tachycardia, depending upon how many are said locally to constitute a paroxysm.

(Ventricular tachycardia: see page 177.)

Should they be reported?

- yes. Not because they require treatment but because they may warn of more serious ventricular dysrhythmias to come.

As expected when you report them, the doctor does not order treatment but asks you to observe closely and report developments. He reminds you that in this hospital, ventricular tachycardia is defined as a sequence of more than nine consecutive ectopic beats occurring at a rate of more than 100 per minute.

A few hours later you observe the following abnormality on the oscilloscope.

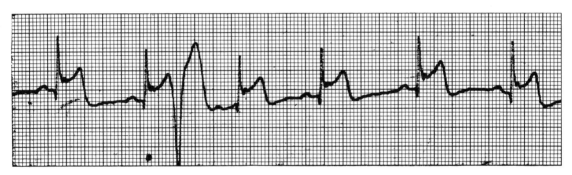

What is it?

- it is an R on T ectopic beat

What is its significance?

- it may initiate ventricular tachycardia or ventricular fibrillation occurring so soon after myocardial infarction

What should you do about it?

- you should report it immediately and prepare suppressive therapy

What suppressive therapy should you prepare?

- a bolus of 100mg lignocaine to be given slowly by intravenous injection over at least two minutes
- this should be followed by a lignocaine infusion of 2mg per minute for 36 hours

(Lignocaine therapy: see page 138.)

Before you have time to start therapy, the ECG changes again.

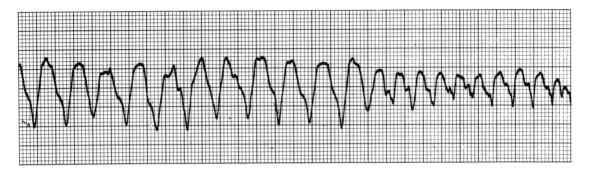

How do you interpret this development?

- as the onset of ventricular tachycardia that appears to be changing into what looks like ventricular fibrillation

What action would you take?

- you should put out a cardiac arrest alarm and start resuscitation immediately

(The treatment of cardiac arrest: see page 128.)

SUMMARY

This was a problem about ventricular ectopic rhythms in acute myocardial infarction. It illustrates the importance of vigilance, so that treatment is confined only to those rhythms that are known to be potentially hazardous to the patient.

Collapse in the Ambulance

A 48 year-old man has collapsed in the ambulance at least five minutes before arriving at the hospital.

In the Admission Department you find that he is pulseless and does not appear to be breathing. You start cardiac resuscitation immediately and summon the doctor on call and the cardiac arrest team.

(The treatment of cardiac arrest: see page 128.)

While waiting for them to arrive, an ECG is recorded.

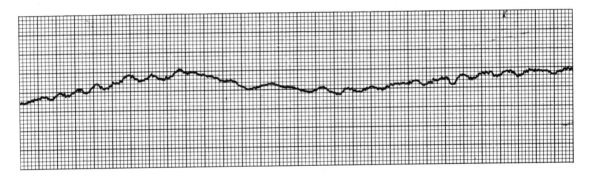

What does it show?

- it shows no evidence of either atrial or ventricular activity and suggests that he has had what is called an asystolic cardiac arrest

(Asystolic arrest: see page 82.)

When the duty registrar arrives a few minutes later, he finds that the patient's pupils are widely dilated and that they do not react to light.

What conclusions can be drawn from this additional piece of information?

- that the patient's brain is already severely damaged

Almost immediately afterwards the cardiac arrest team arrives. What action would you expect them to take?

- they would almost certainly decide that it was too late to attempt resuscitation

The patient has been without effective cardiac output for at least ten minutes and maybe longer. The chances of success are, at best, remote and the brain damage is by now almost certain to be irreversible.

The patient should be regarded as having been brought in dead.

A little later, another patient arrives for admission with a diagnosis of possible myocardial infarction. An ECG is being taken while he is waiting to be seen and he appears to lose consciousness during the recording.

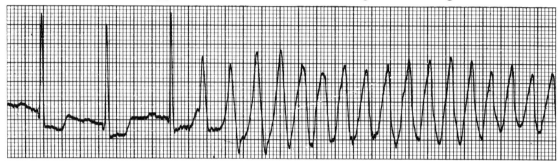

What has happened?

- he has developed ventricular fibrillation

(Ventricular fibrillation: see page 80.)

What action would you take this time?

- the same as before. You should institute immediate cardiac resuscitation and recall the cardiac arrest team.

When the cardiac arrest team arrives, what would you expect them to do this time?

- give an immediate DC shock

(Cardioversion: see pages 130.)

After the shock, his ECG is repeated.

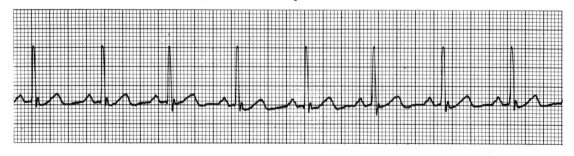

What does it show?

- it shows that the shock has been successful
- he is once again in sinus rhythm

(Sinus rhythm: see page 39.)

What further treatment would you expect them to give before the patient was moved to the ward?

- intravenous sodium bicarbonate (1ml of 8.4% per kg)
- a bolus of 100mg IV lignocaine
- a lignocaine infusion of 2mg per minute

(Lignocaine therapy: see page 138.)

Are any further precautions indicated?

- the journey from the Admission Department to the CCU or emergency ward is notoriously hazardous. He should be accompanied by trained staff with a portable defibrillator so that a further arrest can be dealt with immediately.

SUMMARY

This was a problem about the causes and treatment of cardiac arrest. It illustrates the importance of immediate action and suggests that resuscitation should not be initiated when the signs clearly indicate that it is already too late.

A Patient for Cardioversion

You are sent to relieve in the cardiac emergency ward where a patient with a tachycardia that has failed to respond to drug therapy is about to be cardioverted. Her ECG can be seen on an oscilloscope. The cardiologist who is there to supervise the cardioversion asks for your diagnosis.

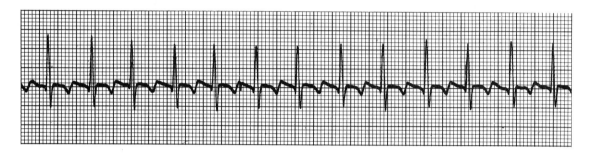

What would you say?

- that it looks like a supraventricular tachycardia; possible atrial flutter with a rapid ventricular response

How could you confirm this diagnosis?

- you suggest that vagal stimulation might make the atrial flutter waves more obvious

He carries out carotid sinus massage. The ECG shows that this has slowed the ventricular rate considerably and the flutter waves are much more obvious.

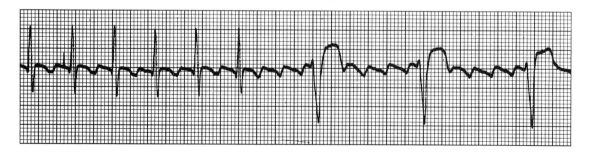

Do you know why this has happened?

- stimulation of the vagus increases the degree of AV block and fewer of the supraventricular stimuli are conducted to the ventricles

(Atrial flutter: see page 62.)

How big a shock should be used to restore normal rhythm?

- usually only a small shock of 25–50 Ws is required to restore normal rhythm in patients with atrial flutter

In this case, 25 Ws is ineffective and 50 Ws produces the change seen below.

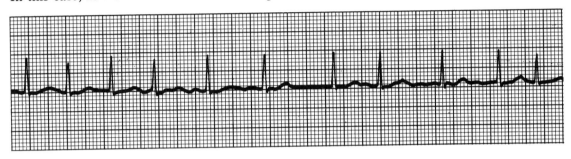

(The treatment of atrial flutter: see page 64. Cardioversion: see page 130.)

What has happened?

- the rhythm has changed to atrial fibrillation

(Atrial fibrillation: see page 59.)

The cardiologist asks:

What do you think should be done now?

- you answer that an attempt should be made to cardiovert the atrial fibrillation to normal sinus rhythm

He agrees and asks:

How much current should be used this time?

- you say that atrial fibrillation is normally much more difficult to convert than atrial flutter and that you have been taught to start with 100 Ws and increase by 100 to a maximum of 400, if necessary

He indicates agreement in principle, but says that because this is clearly a slightly unusual case and that as she has already had two shocks, he is going to give 400 Ws.

Following the 400 Ws the ECG changes again.

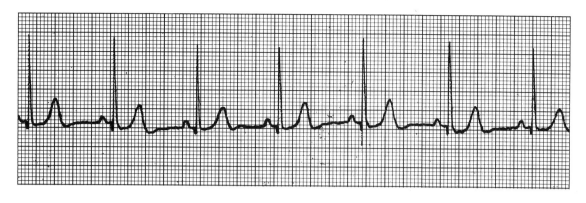

What does it show this time?

- that the third shock has been successful and the patient is back in what appears to be sinus rhythm

(Sinus rhythm: see page 39.)

SUMMARY

This was a problem about the diagnosis and treatment of atrial flutter. It illustrates how vagal stimulation makes the flutter waves more obvious and that DC cardioversion is not always successful with the first shock.

Digitalis Toxicity

An elderly female patient with severe hypertensive heart disease has been taking digoxin and a diuretic for many years because of chronic cardiac failure. After a recent attack of gastro-enteritis, she developed symptoms and signs of digitalis toxicity and has been admitted to hospital for observation and treatment.

Her ECG is being monitored on an oscilloscope, which you have been asked to observe during the night and report any change to the house physician on call. The record when you come on duty is seen below.

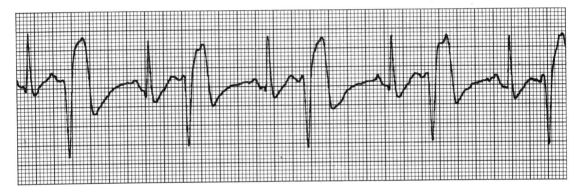

What does it show?

- frequent ventricular ectopic beats

In this case, one ectopic beat occurs after each normal beat, a condition known as coupled rhythm and one that is often seen in patients who have had too much digitalis.

(Ventricular ectopic beats: see page 73.)

What is its significance?

- it almost certainly signifies that the automaticity of the ventricular myocardium has been increased by too much digoxin

(The toxic effects of digoxin: see page 133.)

Some hours later you notice a sudden change in the nature of the ECG.

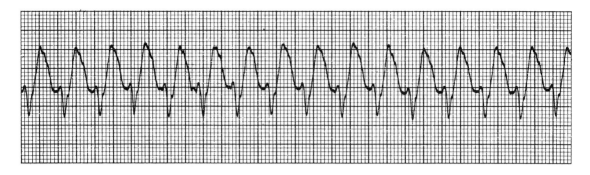

What has happened?

- she has developed ventricular tachycardia

(Ventricular tachycardia: see page 77.)

Would you have reported this abnormality of rhythm if you had been left to use your own discretion?

- yes. It is a serious disorder that should never be ignored.

What is the ventricular rate?

- the ventricular rate is 160 per minute

(Methods of calculating the heart rate are described on pages 10–12.)

Why is it important to count the rate?

- because when you report this change in rhythm to the doctor, he will almost certainly ask what the rate is

Why will he want to know?

- because it will determine whether or not to start treatment

(Therapeutic principles: see page 119.)

In what way will it do this?

- if the rate is very rapid, the paroxysmal tachycardia will have to be brought under control as a matter of urgency

Why do you think this would be necessary?

- because the myocardium is already severely compromised and she will be unable to tolerate a very rapid rate for long without developing acute heart failure

(The effects of disordered action when myocardial function is already poor are discussed on page 37.)

How would you treat such a paroxysm?

216

- normally, it would be terminated with a DC shock and followed by suppressive therapy to prevent a recurrence

In this patient, cardioversion is contra-indicated because the paroxysm is almost certainly due to digitalis toxicity. A DC shock might cause an even more serious disturbance of rhythm, e.g. ventricular fibrillation.

Unfortunately, drug therapy also presents problems in these circumstances. Phenytoin is often effective when used intravenously in the emergency treatment of dysrhythmias caused by digitalis toxicity, but it also tends to depress cardiac function, particularly in the elderly and in patients with heart failure.

(Cardioversion: see page 130. Phenytoin therapy: see page 145.)

Bearing these facts in mind, how do you think they will treat this elderly patient?

- they will probably use lignocaine, remembering that it too must be used with caution in the presence of heart failure

(Lignocaine therapy: see page 138.)

SUMMARY

This was a problem about the diagnosis and treatment of abnormal rhythms caused by the toxic effects of digitalis. It illustrates that many of the methods normally used to treat such abnormalities are not appropriate when the patient has already had too much digoxin.

Index